Handbook of
Sports Medicine
and Science
Alpine Skiing

EDITED BY

Robert E. Leach MD
Department of Orthopaedic Surgery
Boston University Medical School
Boston, Massachusetts

PRINCIPAL CONTRIBUTORS
Daniel Fritschy MD
Department of Surgery
Hôpital Cantonal Universitaire
Geneva
AND
J. Richard Steadman MD
Steadman, Hawkins Clinic
Vail, Colorado

OXFORD

Blackwell Scientific Publications

LONDON EDINBURGH BOSTON

MELBOURNE PARIS BERLIN VIENNA

© 1994 by
Blackwell Scientific Publications
Editorial Offices:
Osney Mead, Oxford OX2 0EL
25 John Street, London WC1N 2BL
23 Ainslie Place, Edinburgh EH3 6AJ
238 Main Street, Cambridge
   Massachusetts 02142, USA
54 University Street, Carlton
   Victoria 3053, Australia

Other Editorial Offices:
Librairie Arnette SA
1, rue de Lille
75007 Paris
France

Blackwell Wissenschafts-Verlag GmbH
Düsseldorfer Str. 38
D-10707 Berlin
Germany

Blackwell MZV
Feldgasse 13
A-1238 Wien
Austria

First published 1994

Set by Excel Typesetters Company, Hong Kong
Printed and bound in Great Britain
at the University Press, Cambridge

DISTRIBUTORS

Marston Book Services Ltd
PO Box 87
Oxford OX2 0DT
(*Orders*: Tel: 0865 791155
          Fax: 0865 791927
          Telex: 837515)

USA
Blackwell Scientific Publications, Inc.
238 Main Street
Cambridge, MA 02142
(*Orders*: Tel: 800 759-6102
           617 876-7000)

Canada
Times Mirror Professional Publishing Ltd
130 Flaska Drive
Markham, Ontario L6G 1B8
(*Orders*: Tel: 800 268-4178
           416 470-6739)

Australia
Blackwell Scientific Publications Pty Ltd
54 University Street
Carlton, Victoria 3053
(*Orders*: Tel: 03 347-5552)

A catalogue record for this title
is available from the British Library

ISBN 0-632-03033-X

Library of Congress
Cataloging-in-Publication Data

Alpine skiing/edited by Robert E. Leach;
   principal contributions, Daniel Fritschy
   and J. Richard Steadman.
         p.   cm. —
   (Handbook of sports medicine and science.)
   Includes index.
   ISBN 0-632-03033-X
      1. Downhill skiing—Physiological aspects.
   2. Sports medicine.   I. Leach, Robert E., 1931–
   II. Fritschy, Daniel.   III. Steadman, J. Richard.
   IV. Series. [DNLM: 1. Skiing—physiology.
   2. Wounds and Injuries—therapy.
   3. Sports Medicine.
   QT 260 A457   1994]
   RC1220.S5A47   1994
   617.1′027—dc20
   DNLM/DLC
   for Library of Congress

Contents

Forewords

It is a pleasure and an honor for me to welcome a new publication by the IOC Medical Commission in this very important year, 1994, during which we shall celebrate the Olympic Centennial and the XVII Olympic Winter Games in Lillehammer, Norway.

After 100 years of existence, the results are positive, and the Olympic Movement goes on growing and occupying an important place in our contemporary society. We have changed and progressed, a great deal and quickly, and the Olympic Movement today has an unprecedented audience and influence. We are well aware of our responsibilities towards athletes and this publication forms part of our manifold and varied response to their needs.

My sincere thanks go to Prince Alexandre de Merode, Chairman of the IOC Medical Commission since 1966, for the impetus he has given to the development of sports medicine sciences and to the establishment of ethical guidelines of health care for athletes.

Juan Antonio Samaranch
IOC President

On behalf of the IOC Medical Commission and its Publications Advisory Sub-Committee, I should like to greet all athletes, coaches, and medical people, and offer them this valuable source of information relative to Alpine skiing.

The International Olympic Committee and its Medical Commission will continue to devote their knowledge and enthusiasm to the cause of scientific research related to human movement and physical activity in sport.

We are certain that the IOC will try to do all that is needed for the improvement and optimization of physical performance through an enhanced understanding of the functioning of the human body. It is our wish and duty to encourage science applied to human movement, physical exercise, and sport.

Prince Alexandre de Merode
Chairman, IOC Medical Commission

Preface and
acknowledgments

I wish to thank the Medical Commission of the International Olympic Committee and, in particular, Prince Alexandre de Merode for support, encouragement, and patience in the production of this handbook.

This handbook would never have made it to publication without the invaluable, always available, and competent assistance of Howard G. Knuttgen. He has toiled long and well for this project.

To Blackwell Scientific Publications Ltd and Mr Peter Saugman go my thanks for unfailing help and expertise.

The principal contributing authors, Dr Daniel Fritschy and Dr J. Richard Steadman, are well known by the international ski world and are well respected by their colleagues and, particularly, by the editor for their excellent contributions to this handbook.

Acknowledgments

The editor wishes to acknowledge the valuable contributions to the production of this handbook of each of the contributing authors listed below. These authors either wrote completely, or contributed significantly to, the chapters which are cited following their names.

Thomas P. Burns MD	Femur
Timothy Foster MD	Functional anatomy
Murray P. Hamlet DVM	Altitude; Cold
Howard G. Knuttgen PhD	Physiology; Nutrition
William Rodkey DVM	Head
Scott L. Sledge MD	Hip
George Thabit MD	Altitude

Robert E. Leach MD
Boston, Massachusetts

Section 1

Introduction

Chapter 1

Basic characteristics of Alpine skiing

Alpine skiing is one of the most exhilarating and pleasurable sports available to us (Fig. 1.1). People can ski from the age of 3 to age 70 and beyond. Skiing in the great outdoors allows us to see beautiful scenery, and visit parts of the world where, under other circumstances, we might not go. It requires great skill to ski well and to race, but skiing skills can develop over a lifetime. On the other hand, with even moderate skill, one can ski competently and safely and enjoy the sport. An attractive aspect of recreational skiing is that the skier usually takes on nature on his or her own terms. One does not have to pick the steepest, most difficult trail on the mountain but can choose trails and areas which are commensurate with one's abilities. Powder, moguls, and open slopes all add to the variety and the potential for enjoyment.

Once we turn to ski racing, however, the skier takes on nature on very different terms.

Skiing is fun, and there are many diverse elements which go into making it fun. Certainly part of it is the thrill of matching wits and physical abilities with nature, but for others the attraction is the excitement of speed which can be attained while skiing. Most people are in some way attracted to speed. Many experience it only vicariously watching car racing, ski racing, etc., on television or in person. For others, this sense of exhilaration is obtained by mechanical means, a car, airplane, or bicycle. In skiing, we achieve speed with the help of the terrain and our equipment and thus experience the exhilaration that this produces. Ski racing is the ultimate in terms of seeking speed, but it is done in a semi-controlled fashion so as to finish the racing course, whether it be slalom, giant slalom, or downhill.

Virtually the only major drawbacks to skiing are the injuries which may be suffered. The risk of injury is enhanced greatly at faster speeds. Fear of injury undoubtedly prevents some people from taking up Alpine skiing, and injuries suffered while skiing will stop others from continuing. Ski racing, whether performed at the top level, such as the World Cup and the Olympics, or at lower levels including schools, colleges, and NASTAR (National Standard Race), is to a

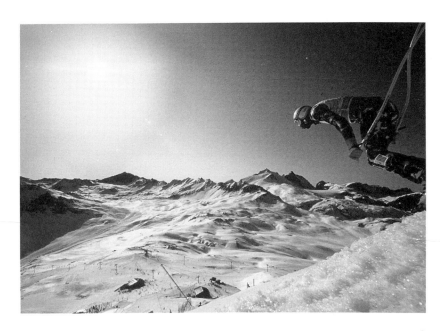

Fig. 1.1 Nature provides spectacular views for Alpine skiing. © Allsport/ C. Cole.

certain extent a conquering of this fear of injury and a controlling of speed. Without question ski racing is potentially more dangerous than normal recreational skiing. However, the skills acquired while ski racing may make recreational skiing even safer for some people.

In this handbook, published by the International Olympic Committee, some of the elements of risk in skiing are examined. This includes the injuries that can occur with skiing, how to deal with them, and, to a lesser extent, how to try to avoid them. A great deal is included here about both the risk of injury and the actual injuries. It must be remembered, however, that skiing has a positive side. It can be conducive to good health. It is an excellent sport for conditioning as it is largely aerobic, although at times with ski racing and fast runs, it becomes anaerobic. Skiing requires one to be in good shape, and doctors frequently advise their patients "to get into shape to ski rather than ski to get into shape." The muscles of the legs, back, and abdomen work in skiing and are made stronger by it. The upper extremities do less, although as everybody knows who has used their ski poles, the first few days on the ski slope can put even the strongest triceps muscle to the test. There is both a heartiness and hardiness to skiers produced by the vigorous physical activity and by being outside. Before going to the substance of this handbook which will deal largely with injuries, it should be made clear that skiing, as a sport, can promote good health.

How dangerous is recreational skiing? In one of the first ski injury studies completed in 1961 at Sun Valley, Idaho (Tapper, 1978), it was determined that, at that time, the rate of injury was 7.4 per 1000 skier days. In 1976, 15 years later, another study found in the same area that the injury rate had fallen to 2.6 injuries per 1000 skier days. Recreational skiing has become safer.

What factors contributed to this dramatic fall in the injury rate? Most observers point to the use of better equipment, particularly safety bindings, which are now better manufactured and adjusted. Most good ski bindings now in use, release both at the heel and at the toe, and can release at multiple angles with torque at the toe. Binding adjustment is a critical factor in promoting safer skiing. Bindings should be adjusted for the individual skier for his or her height, weight, skill and, in some instances, for the conditions which

the skier is to face. For the recreational skier, it is likely that binding adjustments are best performed by the professionals working in ski shops. For the racing skier, binding adjustments are performed both by the racers and by the people with whom they work. In various studies about ski injuries, one of the most frequently mentioned factors concerning the cause of ski injuries is that many skiers tighten down their bindings following a previous fall from which the skier has released. This tightening of the binding may then lead to a situation where the leg does not release during a fall and a subsequent injury will occur.

Bindings are not the only equipment which have experienced radical change in skiing. Skis, boots, and poles have all been improved during the past several decades. Skis, particularly for the recreational skiers, are shorter, have better edges, and are much easier to turn and control. Ski boots have seen a major change. They are higher and stiffer and thus transmit bodily movements to the skis more rapidly and accurately, which allows people to have better edge control and to ski better. The combination of better skis and boots have made it much easier to be in control and not to fall. There is an old but serviceable axiom which states that, "if you do not fall, you do not get hurt skiing." About the only time that axiom does not hold is when you collide with another skier or a stationary object. Unfortunately, ski racing or high speeds may be the cause of such collision injuries. The obvious way for the recreational skier or racer to avoid problems is to gain better control, which is a product of skill and equipment.

Equipment has modified injury statistics. The stiff, higher boots have dramatically changed the pattern of ski injuries. The incidence of ankle sprains and fractures has gone down, as has the incidence of tibial fractures; however, a higher percentage of knee injuries is now found. The high boot has been very useful in helping people to use their edges in skiing more effectively but has not been kind to the knee.

While equipment changes have been the key element in helping to reduce injuries both for the recreational and racing skier, other factors have also contributed to the decreased injury rate for the recreational skier. The grooming and correct marking of ski slopes throughout the world has become immeasurably better. Marking trails as expert, intermediate, or novice has made it possible for all skiers to pick a slope commensurate with their own ability. It is now easier to ski on these slopes and the risk of a fall or unexpected encounter has decreased.

One factor which remains a major problem is particularly germane for the readers of this book. The faster one goes in skiing the more likely one is to experience an injury. As speed increases the injuries suffered are proportionately more severe. Ski racing speeds have increased tremendously in the last several decades. This seems to be a combination of the ski racers themselves and better equipment; with equipment being a large factor. Since speed is an objective of the ski racer, it becomes incumbent upon the racer to have pinpoint control and thus avoid most injuries.

The purpose of this handbook is to bring basic information to ski racers, coaches, and medical people who deal with ski racers. The causes and treatments of a multitude of injuries that can be suffered while ski racing will be discussed, plus certain other medical problems, such as exposure to cold, sun, and high altitudes which may result from being on the ski slopes while racing. The reader is also provided with the basics of physiology and anatomy concerning ski racing which, when added to the section on training, should be helpful to anybody concerned with ski racing. The recommended reading lists will show other sources of information for those who want to explore certain topics in more depth.

Reference

Tapper, E.M. (1978) Ski injuries from 1939 to 1976. The Sun Valley experience. *Am. J. Sports Med.* **6**:114–121.

Chapter 2

Clothing

While discussing clothing as it relates to ski racing, certain problems must be recognized. At the very top of the ski racing contingent will be the World Cup and professional racing skiers with their sleek helmets and form-fitting one-piece outfits, which help to decrease wind resistance and thus increase speed. On a cold, windy day, the skier wearing that outfit for a brief period of time loses much body heat; however, given the circumstances, with outer clothing available before and after racing plus people to help with redressing, the skier is not at any real risk. Usually ski racing is performed under circumstances quite different from these, and there are many factors which must be considered with regard to clothing. Protection, comfort, cost, and for many, lastly, the effect on speed should be considered (Fig. 2.1).

Helmets should be worn by ski racers. Helmets do not guarantee that a racer will not suffer a head or neck injury. However, they will protect skiers from many head injuries and may make a potentially more serious injury into a lesser one. Helmets must be well-fitted to be effective and should have a face guard component. Cost becomes a problem, particularly in the younger ski racer, and many people competing in lower levels of competition may not be wearing helmets. In the same way that using a seatbelt in a car decreases the injury rate the use of a helmet decreases the injury rate in ski racing. For younger children, helmets can be a problem because of their weight as the neck of a child is not strong, and the child may not be able to wear a particular helmet comfortably (Fig. 2.2).

The next consideration for most skiers and ski racers is protection from the cold. Most skiing, including ski racing is performed in cold weather. The concepts are well known. Dress in multiple layers with a water- and wind-resistant or water-repellent outer shell which helps to trap the warm air created by our bodies between the clothing layers, and by so doing, we insulate our bodies and retain heat. The ability to stay warm on a ski slope is controlled by the body's ability to produce heat which must then be trapped in an envelope around the body. Large amounts of heat are lost from the head and neck area, and thus the skier must cover the head and protect the neck. The more of the head that is covered by a cap, particularly a woolen cap, the more heat is retained. The outer jacket should close up tightly at the neck to retain body heat. At the sleeve, there should be Velcro or some other device which will keep the sleeves tight so that snow does not get in thus causing heat loss.

During the exercise of ski racing, heat and perspiration are produced under the clothing. Problems may arise when there are several runs during an afternoon. During the warm-up and a race, the skier may start

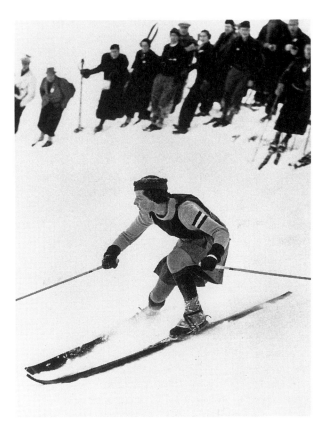

Fig. 2.1 Competitors in the 1936 Winter Olympic Games did not use protective equipment and employed bindings that could cause injury. © CIO.

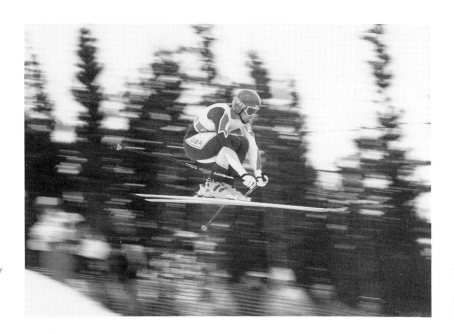

Fig. 2.2 Participants in contemporary events have the benefit of equipment designed for both speed and safety. © Sports Illustrated.

sweating and then care must be taken not to cool down too much as this may increase the risk of mild hypothermia or even muscle stiffness. Wool is an excellent fabric to use because it absorbs moisture and still retains heat. Cotton absorbs moisture and can be used next to the skin. The racer who has to wait around after having exercised must be concerned about the possibility of losing body heat.

Frequently, skiers protect the upper body better than they do the legs. If some type of undergarment is not worn on the legs, heat loss can be extensive. The combination of cotton or thermal long johns, ski pants, and an outer ski garment keeps one toasty! This is probably the preferred clothing for the recreational skier, but the racer would find this bulky. The key is to dress for the cold and if the clothes are taken off for the race, they must be immediately available for protection afterwards.

Hands and feet present a special problem since they are at the distal end of the body's circulation and heat production, and with a large surface area, they tend to lose heat easily. Also, they do not themselves produce much heat. Mittens are warmer than gloves, but most racers will use gloves. It helps to have the proper choice of an insulating fabric in the glove, and by using an inner light-weight cotton or silk glove, some heat is retained. The tighter the glove, the more likely one is to have cold hands, but if it is only for a short

period of time during ski racing, this is unlikely to be a major problem. Boots are more properly described in Chapter 3. However, most people do agree that the combination of one light pair of socks and one pair of woolen socks is the best way to keep your feet warm and dry for skiing. Boots with an attached heater pack are a further step along the way to comfort.

The outer garments should be if not water resistant, then at least water repellant. The fabric should breath, which is why some of the new fabrics have become so popular. They stop the wind and moisture from getting in while still trapping air inside and allowing a little ventilation so as to avoid the effect of a rubber suit in a sauna. All skiers recognize that wind is a major factor in producing wind chill. The more wind there is, the more insulation and clothing is needed and the wind-resistant outer shell becomes mandatory.

The 1–3 min of a ski race are not a huge problem in terms of being cold. However, all racers must dress warmly before and after the race and not allow themselves to become cold, particularly as they are preparing for future runs. For a skier ascending the racing ladder, the streamlining effect of clothing becomes progressively more important, and by that time, hopefully he or she has accumulated experience in learning how to dress and briefly strip down to the essentials for racing.

Chapter 3

Equipment

Equipment is a critical aspect of ski racing. While clothing and the use of helmets for racing have been discussed in Chapters 1 and 2, skis, poles, boots, and bindings have not yet been covered. With regard to skis and poles, anybody who is interested in ski racing should have access to information from coaches, other racers, ski magazines, and ski shops which would enable the racer to make the proper choice of skis and poles. The same information resources are available for ski boots. There is, however, one important point to make with regard to ski boots and that is that the ski boots must fit from the very beginning. One does not break in ski boots. If they need any modifications to fit the foot well, this should be completed before leaving the shop and starting to ski. Otherwise, problems with the feet are inevitable and a constant battle to try to reshape the boots may be the result.

With regard to equipment, nothing is more important than the bindings and some type of safety bindings are required. There are a variety of bindings for sale and a great deal of literature is available both in ski magazines and even in medical journals. Any binding being used in ski racing should have both a heel and toe upward release plus the usual side-to-side releases available at the toe for all angles. No recommendations are presented regarding any particular bindings because there is information available to help with this choice and because bindings change from year to year. It is recommended that you choose a modern, near top of the line type of binding. What is certain is that all bindings must be kept in perfect working order. They must be adjusted for the particular skier and for his or her skill and for the conditions to be entered. Anybody who is in ski racing should know enough about bindings to adjust their own bindings properly. It is recommended that skiers attend a workshop course under the standards of the American Society for Testing and Materials (ASTM) and in the usual circumstances, racers should use normal ASTM shop practices for their bindings. One of the major problems is the tendency for all ski racers to tighten their bindings down beyond the usual recommended standards. Skiers at the very top level will undoubtedly set their bindings tighter than is preferable. However, a strong recommendation is made that ski racers follow the usual recommended binding settings to help to avoid injury.

Recommended reading

Tapper, E.M. (1978) Ski injuries from 1939 to 1976. The Sun Valley experience. *Am. J. Sports Med.* **6**:114–121.

Section 2

Biological Foundations

Chapter 4

Functional anatomy

Alpine skiing requires a complex interaction between the central nervous system and the skeletal muscles of both the upper and lower extremities plus concise control of the body. When one progresses from Alpine skiing as a recreational sport into racing, the interaction and the precision demanded between the various parts of the body and the brain becomes even more intricate. Control over the skeletal muscles and the joints which they interact with, allows the skier to move quickly, turn precisely, and maintain his or her body equilibrium.

During the 1990s, it is obvious that the techniques, equipment, and even the terrain upon which competitive Alpine skiing is performed have changed dramatically. Competition has become more intense and as both the equipment and skiers have improved, the velocities reached by today's racers are well above those seen 25 years ago. Racers now reach speeds in the 97 and 113 km/h (60 and 70 mile/h) range, a dramatic increase over 30 years ago, and this puts a premium on the skier to maintain control, both to win and to avoid injury.

These higher speeds, changes in the equipment and terrain, and some technique improvements, have resulted in unusual demands being placed on the skier's musculoskeletal system. To understand and ultimately prevent the injuries of the élite skier, basic anatomy and kinesiology as it pertains to skiing and ski racing must be understood. The forces acting upon the skiers as well as the forces which the skier generates must also be recognized.

In this chapter, the basic anatomy of the upper and lower extremity as it pertains to skiing will be discussed and the natural forces acting upon the élite skier will be briefly analysed. This is followed by a discussion of the kinesiology and applied anatomy as it relates to Alpine skiing.

Basic anatomy

Ankle

Although the ankle joint is injured far less frequently than formerly because of the advent of the stiff boot, it still remains a very important joint in the mechanics of skiing and is still subject to injury. The ankle joint is composed of three different bones: the tibia, the talus, and the fibula. The medial malleolus is the medial and distal termination of the tibia. The lateral malleolus is the distal portion of the fibula and the talus is the small bone which sits between the medial and lateral malleolus. Strong ligaments medially and laterally hold the talus in place acting against any forces which would displace them.

There are very strong, short ligaments which prevent the tibia and the fibula from separating which are termed the syndesmotic ligaments. Most ankle fractures involve the distal fibula but at the same time, there may or may not be a tear of the medial deltoid and the syndesmotic ligaments between the tibia and the fibula. The more ligaments that are torn, the more severe is the injury suffered. In some major injuries, not only may the fibula be broken but the medial malleolus may be broken rather than the medial ligaments. With the high, stiff boots now worn, the incidence of ankle fractures and ligamentous injuries to the ankle has markedly declined.

Lower leg

The lower leg has two bones, the larger of which is called the tibia, and the smaller is the fibula. The fibula is a rather narrow bone which transmits only 10% of the weight of the body. The tibia, a much larger bone, transmits most of the body weight. These two bones are surrounded by muscles, although the anterior portion of the tibia is subcutaneous and thus more readily available to injury including contusions. The muscles of the lower leg are divided into three compartments.
1 The anterior compartment which contains the muscles controlling the ankle and toe dorsiflexors.
2 The lateral compartment which overlies the fibula contains the muscles which evert the foot.
3 The posterior compartment muscles which control the ability to plantarflex the foot and toes and to turn the foot in.

During skiing, the effect of most of these muscles is relatively minimal due to the immobilization of the ankle within the ski boot. The subcutaneous location of the tibia makes it prone to injury and with the high, stiff ski boot, there is a "stress riser" produced on the tibia at the junction of the boot and the bone. Where the boot ends, the bone must now absorb a large amount of pressure which can predispose to a fracture, i.e. the boot top fracture.

Knee

The knee is under great stress during Alpine skiing and racing and severe ligamentous injuries in competitive skiers are almost epidemic in nature. The knee is composed of three bones (Fig. 4.1): the femur (the large bone of the thigh), the tibia, and the patella (the knee cap). The knee can be divided into three compartments which helps to understand the anatomy easier. The patellofemoral compartment contains the patella and the femur. There is articular cartilage on the undersurface of the patella which glides against the articular cartilage of the femur. A groove on the femur helps the patella to slide back and forth as the knee goes from flexion to extension and back. With the knee straight there is virtually no contact between the patella and the femur. However, when the knee reaches about 30° of flexion, the patella begins to slide into the groove on the femur and continues this until somewhat past 90° of flexion.

The articular surfaces of the joint form a very slippery surface. In fact, the coefficient of friction between these two gliding surfaces is a quarter of the coefficient of friction of ice gliding upon ice. Therefore,

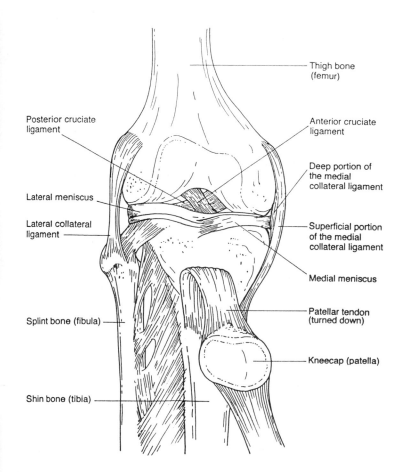

Thigh bone
(femur)

Posterior cruciate
ligament

Anterior cruciate
ligament

Deep portion of
the medial
collateral ligament

Lateral meniscus

Lateral collateral
ligament

Superficial portion
of the medial
collateral ligament

Medial meniscus

Splint bone (fibula)

Patellar tendon
(turned down)

Kneecap (patella)

Shin bone (tibia)

Fig. 4.1 The knee joint (anterior aspect, right knee).

anything causing irregularity of the articular surface of the patellofemoral joint causes problems on the undersurface of the knee cap and that may cause pain, clicking, and further damage to the articular cartilage.

The medial compartment of the knee is composed of articular surfaces of the tibia and the femur and contains the medial meniscus (commonly called the medial cartilage) plus the medial collateral ligament. The medial meniscus is composed of fibrocartilage and is attached to the outside of the tibia through small ligaments. The meniscus is shaped similar to a C and sits on top of the tibia acting as a shock absorber to cushion the compression of the femoral surface against the tibia. It also in some ways, acts as a restraint to help limit the motion of the tibia and the femur.

What is termed the medial collateral ligament is actually composed of several different ligaments along the medial aspect of the knee joint plus the posterior medial knee capsule. The medial collateral ligament prevents side-to-side and angular translation of the tibia on the femur as well as helping to prevent some anterior translation. The medial collateral ligament is exceedingly prone to injury when the inside ski edge is caught in the snow which causes external rotation and stress to the knee (i.e. the lower leg angles away from the midline of the body).

The lateral compartment is composed of the articular surfaces of the femur and the tibia as well as the lateral meniscus and the lateral ligament complex. The lateral meniscus is similar to the medial meniscus, although it is even more C-shaped and acts in the same manner as the medial meniscus.

The lateral collateral ligament complex contains the distinct lateral collateral ligament as well as a posterior thickening of the capsule which is termed the arcuate complex. There is also a small popliteus tendon which goes from the femur down posteriorly slanting towards its attachment behind the tibia. This lateral collateral ligament, arcuate complex, and the popliteus tendon, all help to prevent varus stress and also help prevent translation of the tibia forward on the femur. (Varus is when the lower leg is angled in towards the midline of the body.)

Between the medial and lateral compartment lies the intercondylar notch. This notch contains two ligaments which are of great importance to the skier and to any athlete. The anterior cruciate ligament (ACL) is composed of several fiber bundles which are attached to the anteromedial surface of the tibia and extend up to the lateral femoral condyle posteriorly. This very strong and important ligament prevents anterior translation of the tibia on the femur and subsequent instability of the knee. The posterior cruciate ligament lies behind the ACL and crosses in the opposite direction of the ACL and is attached to the posterior tibia and the medial femoral condyle. The posterior cruciate ligament is a large, strong ligament which prevents posterior translation of the tibia on the femur. The design of the knee is an engineering nightmare which allows excellent mobility with relatively good stability. However, when large forces are applied to the knee the strength of the various ligamentous complexes can be overcome and the structural integrity of the knee and the ligaments can be compromised. When the ligamentous anatomy of the knee is compromised the knee does not function well and secondary injury to the menisci and the articular cartilage may be possible. At the same time, there may be a primary injury to the menisci and even to the joint surfaces as the result of trauma from skiing.

Thigh

The thigh has only one bone, the femur, which is the strongest and largest bone in the human body. It is completely surrounded by a large mass of skeletal muscle. The skeletal muscle mass can be again divided into three different compartments. The anterior compartment contains the quadriceps muscles which are the muscles responsible for extending the knee by virtue of their attachment to the patella and to the anterior portion of the tibia below the knee. The quadriceps muscles are dynamic stabilizers of the knee joint and by their contraction may help to prevent excess rotation and abnormal movement of the tibia on the femur.

The posterior compartment muscles are the hamstrings which include the semi-tendinosus, semi-membranosus, and the biceps femoris. The hamstrings act to flex the knee and they also are dynamic stabilizers of the knee. The semi-tendinosus and semi-membranosus help to stabilize the medial aspect while the biceps femoris goes to the lateral side and is a stabilizer there. Strengthening of the hamstring muscles can be very helpful in the absence of the ACL because the hamstrings work synergistically with the ACL in preventing anterior translation of the tibia on the femur.

The medial compartment muscles originate from the pelvis and insert on the medial and distal portions of the femur and tibia. These muscles are strong and provide adduction of the lower extremity (adduction, pulls the leg towards the midline of the body). Adductors are very powerful in skiers and skaters and are necessary to bring the skis together to execute precise and beautiful turns.

Hip

The hip joint is a ball and socket joint. The socket is the acetabulum and the ball is the femoral head. The hip joint is designed to have nearly unlimited motion although the strong ligaments surrounding the hip do prevent more than 90° of abduction, i.e. motion away from the midline of the body. The hip joint is exceedingly stable because of the deep socket and the size of the femoral head. The anterior ligaments of the hip prevent a posterior dislocation. There are large muscles which surround the hip and which help to control the movement and stabilize the hip. The gluteal muscles are strong abductors and extensors of the hip joint. These muscles attach to the pelvis and insert on the lateral aspect of the proximal femur. There are short external rotators which attach to the posterior pelvis and proximal femur. The short rotators act to rotate the hip externally. The iliopsoas muscle arises from the pelvis and the lower lumbar spine and attaches to the medial aspect of the proximal femur and is the most powerful flexor of the hip.

Upper extremity

The upper extremity and the trunk are less important in skiing and ski injuries than the lower extremity. They are, however, important in a variety of ways and are becoming increasingly more subject to injury. In the upper extremity the two most important areas subject to injury are the shoulder and the thumb.

Shoulder

The shoulder is another ball and socket joint, although very different from the hip joint in that it allows an al-

most complete freedom of movement to the shoulder. This allows the hand to be positioned in space almost anywhere relative to the body. The socket is called the glenoid and is relatively small and shallow compared to the socket of the hip joint. The head of the humerus is held in this socket by virtue of ligamentous structures which are not nearly as strong as those around the hip and by the muscle tendon units which attach around the shoulder. Because of the small socket and relatively weak ligaments holding the head in the socket, the shoulder is easily subject to injury and to the possibility of dislocation, i.e. going out of joint. At the same time, it does have excellent mobility which allows for all the motions that one needs.

Thumb

A strong and mobile thumb (Fig. 4.2) is essential for normal function of the hand. The thumb is able to flex, extend, adduct/abduct, and oppose (the action of bringing the distal tip of the thumb against the distal tip of the finger). This mobility occurs because of the synchronous action of the metacarpophalangeal joint and the oddly shaped carpometacarpal joint (saddle-shaped), which is where the motion for opposition occurs. The ligaments at the carpometacarpal joint are strong and seldom injured. However, in skiing, while holding the ski pole or falling on the outstretched hand, great stress can be applied to the ulnar collateral ligament which is attached at the base of the proximal phalanx of the thumb and head of the metacarpal. This ligament keeps the thumb from being forced away from the fingers as would occur in the act of pinching between the thumb and index finger. The adductor pollicis muscle aponeurosis overlies the ulnar ligament and when the ligament is torn, the aponeurosis may become interposed between the ligament ends and prevent healing of the ligament.

Forces

There are many forces which act upon the skier and, in fact, the performance of the skier is determined by these natural forces plus those exerted by the skier. An understanding of these forces may allow the skier to modify technique and to enhance performance and to avoid injury.

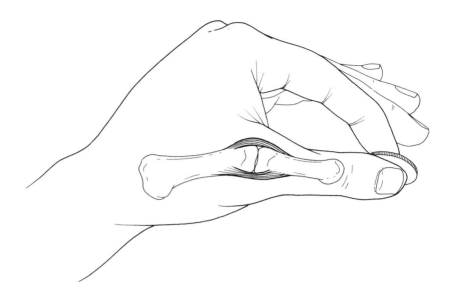

Fig. 4.2 The thumb (left hand).

Weight of the skier

The weight of the skier acts in a vertical and downward direction through the skier's own center of gravity. By adding small increments of weight, if one were in a frictionless environment, the velocity of the skier could be theoretically increased. The key here is, of course, that we are not in a frictionless environment.

Ground reaction force

There is a force that the ground, i.e. the snow, exerts upon the skier via the skis and to a much less extent, the poles. The skier uses this ground reaction force to his or her advantage to make turns and at the same time tries to decrease some of this force by the sliding surface of the skis and by waxes added to the skis.

Air resistance

Air resistance force increases as the magnitude of velocity of the skier increases. The skier may counteract this force by flexing the hips, knees, and ankles and putting the body into a tucked racing position so that air resistance is decreased and theoretically downhill speed is increased.

Basic kinesiology

If one were to view a video tape of an élite skier and show the speed of the tape down, several distinct phases could be identified. The following is a brief synopsis of the phases and the forces which act upon the skier during each phase.

Phase 1: the crouch phase

This phase is characterized by the skier advancing straight down the slope. The center of gravity of the skier is low, located directly above an imaginary line passing vertically between the inside edges of the skis and slightly forward to the ankle joints. The skis are equally weighted. The hips, knees, and ankles are flexed which allows for the regulation of undesirable upward movement of the skis caused by aberrations in the terrain. There is a forward inclination of the torso and upper extremities which allows for decreased wind resistance and a decrease in the down reaction force. With the hips, knees and ankles flexed, there is a tendency for the skis to shoot out from underneath the skier. The forward position of the skier allows for the center of gravity to be positioned anterior to the ankle and therefore helps to alleviate the tendency to fall backward.

The medial and lateral collateral ligaments of the knee are not under stress during this phase and the cruciate ligaments are also not in danger. The posterior leg muscles and the hamstrings are active during this phase to help flex the knee and to prevent anterior translation of the tibia on the femur.

At this point there are no rotary forces acting on the torso or the upper extremities. Difficulties during this phase can occur with sudden decelerations such as when the skier goes over an obstruction or a bump. The deceleration causes a sudden extension of the knees with stress applied to the ACL to prevent forward translation of the tibia on the femur. If this deceleration force exceeds the tensile strength of the ACL, a tear may occur. If a rotational stress is placed on the knee along with the deceleration force, there may be injury to either of the collateral ligaments and the menisci.

Phase 2: turn initiation phase

This phase commences when the skier reaches the first turning point such as a gate. It is characterized by the skier making a turn from the crouched position. In order to execute the turn, the skier plants his or her pole ahead of, but generally along side, the weighted downhill skier. The skier exerts a downward force on the pole which assists in extension of the hips, knees, and ankles. This causes the center of gravity to move upward and forward compared to the previous phase. The skier then thrusts the heels in the direction required to make the turns as the body is coming up. To maintain balance the skier must offset this heel motion with some rotation of the torso in the opposite direction of the turns. The turn has now started.

Phase 3: turn execution stage

This phase is characterized by the ski edges cutting the snow and literally holding the skier along the required track. There is an increase in the weight of the skier on the downhill ski and an increase in the ground reactive force. The center of gravity once again shifts to a lower position as the hips and knees flex. The downhill ski is weighted and is more prone to injury if a ski edge or tip is caught. If the inside edge of the ski is caught a valgus force is thrust upon the knee, thereby stressing the medial collateral ligament. If this force continues, the medial collateral ligament and eventually the anterior cruciate and medial meniscus are at risk of injury, particularly if the ski does not lift from the snow or if the leg and foot does not release quickly from its binding.

Phase 4: exit from the turn

This phase begins as the skier clears the turn or exits the gate. The skier plants the pole lifting the weight from the skis and again using a heel thrust and with some counter-rotation of the torso, this propels the skier straight downhill as the next gate is approached. The center of gravity rises as the hips and knees extend somewhat and ground force reaction decreases as the skier is lifting the weight from the skis.

In ski racing all of these motions are done more quickly and energetically and yet because they are done more smoothly, they are more difficult to follow. As the speed increases, all of the forces that are acting increase and thus the potential for injury increases with the speed. It is only the skill of the racer which prevents injury happening more frequently. With the new equipment, increased speed, and the more demanding race conditions, more severe injuries are occurring.

Chapter 5

Physiology

The Alpine skier is delivered to a particular altitude by means of a mechanical lift which requires an investment of energy to run the lift and elevate the skier. The ski racer and the ski equipment then represent potential energy relative to their collective mass (kg) and the difference between the race start altitude and the race finish altitude on the mountain (i.e. the vertical drop). In Fig. 5.1, the skier with a combined body and equipment mass of 80 kg will be attracted toward the center of the earth by a force (gravity) that would cause a downward acceleration of 9.8 m/s if the skier could engage in free fall with no air resistance. There would be vertical or downward movement only.

In the example, the potential energy for the skier and equipment can be calculated as the total mass (80 kg) multiplied by the force of the earth's gravity (9.8 N/kg) multiplied by the potential change in altitude (900 m). The calculation results in a potential energy of the skier and equipment at the start of 705 600 J (or 705.6 kJ or 168.6 kcal).

However, the Alpine skier races downward on a course that has a forward or horizontal component as well. The skier will encounter resistance to forward movement because of the friction involved in the ski : snow interface and because of the fluid resistance of the air through which the skier moves. Additionally, the skier is required to turn in order to pass through the gates of the race course. Each turn involves a more forceful ski-to-snow interface and, therefore, significantly more resistance to forward movement. The greater both the number and tightness of the turns are, the greater is the resistance to the skier's velocity. The longer the length of the course per meter of vertical drop, the greater is the total force of resistance relative to gravitational force and the slower is the progression of the skier.

All of the potential energy that can be calculated for the skier, as in the example, has been lost as the skier crosses the finish line and stops. It is dissipated in the form of energy lost to friction and air resistance. In both cases, the velocity of the skier can be increased if the ski-to-snow friction and the air resistance are reduced.

If it is assumed that the skier was a male competitor of average size with a maximal oxygen uptake of 60 ml/kg and that the race demanded at least 90% of maximal aerobic power for 100 s, it can be calculated that the total metabolic energy cost of the race to the skier would be approximately 170 kJ (40 kcal). As described above, it cost 705.6 kJ of energy to elevate the skier to the start and, if the skier had climbed to this height, the metabolic cost to the skier would have been minimally 3000 kJ. The relatively low value of 170 kJ for the race represents the metabolic energy

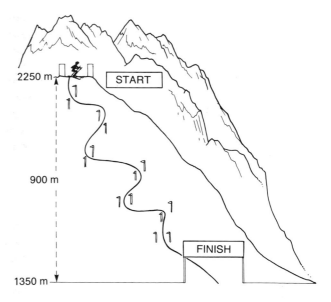

Mass of skier + equipment = 80 kg

Force of earth's gravity = 9.8 N × 80 = 784 N

Vertical drop of race course = 900 m

Potential energy of skier + equipment =

    784 N × 900 m = 705 600 J =

    705.6 kJ = 168.6 kcal

Metabolic cost of a downhill run = 167 000 J = 167 kJ = 40 kcal

Fig. 5.1 Energetic considerations of a skier engaged in a downhill event.

cost of the skier controlling the descent caused by gravitational pull downward so as to follow the race course.

These energy considerations are related to the physics of completing a race course in the fastest possible time. The biological or metabolic energy cost to the skier will be determined by the forces required of the skier's skeletal muscles to complete the turns and maintain balance during the race. Concerning the biologic aspects of Alpine skiing, a review is presented in this chapter of the mechanisms of force and power development by muscles, the energy requirements of the force and power development, and the involvement of the body's physiologic support systems of respiration and circulation in the total process.

Alpine race courses

The traditional disciplines in Alpine ski racing are the downhill, the super G, the giant slalom, and the slalom. The events differ from each other in distance, total number of gates, distance between gates, and the speeds of progression of the skiers (see Table 5.1).

The downhill course is the longest and usually involves a lower number of gates. It is, therefore, characterized by large turns and high speeds. Competitive events involve a single run.

The slalom is at the other extreme and comprises the shortest course with the largest number of gates

per course length. Therefore, this event is characterized by very tight turns and the lowest speeds of progression. The order of finish for the competitors is determined by two runs on separate courses.

The giant slalom involves a longer course than the slalom with a smaller number of gates per course length. Therefore, the courses follow a more open line, the turns are less tight, and the velocities are greater than the slalom. Two runs on separate courses are also employed for this discipline.

The super G is a hybrid of giant slalom and downhill. The turns are not as tight as in the giant slalom and the course in longer. Speeds are attained which are intermediate to the giant slalom and downhill. The order of finish is determined by one run.

The data presented in Table 5.1, as representative of a typical international competition, present vivid evidence of the physiologic demands on the skiers competing in the different events. It can be observed that, while the course lengths are shorter in each case for women, the differences among the four events are relatively comparable to the course lengths for men. Comparing the extremes of the downhill event and the slalom for either gender, the lengths of the courses and the density of gates result in greater than a two-fold difference in speed. Downhill skiers attain speeds in the range of 22–29 m/s, which translate into 80–105 km/h or 50–65 mile/h. The number of gates does not differ greatly between the two events and,

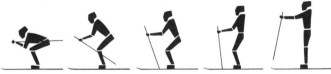

Table 5.1 Alpine ski race courses – representative data for a typical competition. Specifications for each event are regulated by national and international regulations as related to minimum and maximum requirements for such features as vertical drop and number of gates

Course	Vertical drop (m)	Length (m)	No. of gates	Av. speed of winner (m/s)	Av. distance between gates
Men's downhill	973	3048	42	27.6	72.6
Women's downhill	878	2770	40	24.4	69.2
Men's super G	535	1650	39	22.5	42.3
Women's super G	498	1510	45	18.6	33.6
Men's giant slalom	384	1450	47	17.2	30.8
Women's giant slalom	398	1320	45	15.3	29.3
Men's slalom	220	530	65	12.2	8.2
Women's slalom	190	480	52	10.5	9.2

NB A skier makes two runs for competition in the giant slalom and slalom events with total elapsed time determining finish order.

therefore, the tightness of the turns and the emphasis on both strength and quickness of movement is much greater for the slalom. The super G and giant slalom lie intermediate in these respects.

The race characteristics have important implications for the conditioning of the body muscles, particularly of the thigh and lower leg. The longer the race, the longer the intervals during which a racer holds a crouched position. The shorter the event and the tighter the turns, the greater the demand for high strength and high power performed rapidly and in quick succession.

All events in Alpine skiing share certain characteristics when compared with other competitive sports. The Alpine events are of relatively short duration, with a typical race lasting between 40 s (slalom) and 115 s (downhill). Compared to running events, this would place Alpine skiing in the range between a 400- and an 800-m run. Both of the running events are highly anaerobic in terms of the generation of energy for the muscular performance.

Important differences between running and Alpine skiing involve the fact that the runners' leg muscles are contracting for briefer intervals in order to maintain 110–120 double-strides·min^{-1}. Additionally, the runner elevates body mass with each stride which emphasizes concentric muscle actions. The skier's muscle actions, especially in the super G and downhill, are much longer and slower and, in all Alpine disciplines, the emphasis is on eccentric muscle actions as the skier opposes the downward pull of gravity. The runner's muscles are engaged in very brief eccentric actions with the foot strike of the lead leg while the Alpine skiers muscles are involved in somewhat slower eccentric actions of longer duration during each turn, particularly in the downhill and super G.

The physiological challenge

The description of the demands of a particular sports performance begins with an assessment of the muscular activity involved. Events requiring long-term endurance require less of the muscles in terms of the force and power development but emphasize the availability of the energy-yielding compounds of carbohydrate and fat and the constant delivery of oxygen over a long period of time. Events of great strength and power require much larger muscle mass and the specificity of conditioning the muscles for the production of high forces.

The muscles depend on the other systems of the body for proper functioning. The digestive system provides the nutrients to the blood stream. The circulatory system delivers these nutrients plus oxygen to the muscle cells. Carbon dioxide is taken from the tissues to the lungs. Additionally, the blood circulates hormones and plays a major role in temperature regulation. The respiratory system interacts with the circulatory system to provide oxygen and eliminate carbon dioxide.

The story begins with muscle.

Skeletal muscles

Skeletal muscles, also referred to as voluntary muscles, are those of which we are consciously aware and able to control. They attach to and cause movement of the body skeleton. The principal unit of organization in each muscle is a long, cylindrical cell which is commonly called the muscle fiber. Muscle fibers do not function independently within an individual muscle but are coordinated by a network of nerve cells emanating from the central nervous system.

A single muscle is composed of thousands of muscle fibers together with supporting connective tissue, blood vessels, and nerve fibers. The number of muscle fibers contained in each muscle varies considerably and depends on the size and function of the particular muscle. Each fiber has an outer membrane which encloses a gelatin-like sarcoplasm, the protein filaments that develop the force and power, and energy-producing units that are essential for human movement. The electron micrograph presented in Fig. 5.2 provides a view of the interior of a muscle fiber and shows the contractile proteins (actin and myosin), the energy-generating units (mitochondria), and the storage of the primary fuel (glycogen) for the performance of Alpine skiing.

Although the precise mechanisms for producing the force in an active muscle fiber are not fully understood, it is commonly held that, when a fiber is activated, the actin and myosin filaments attempt to slide past each other, thus shortening the length of the fiber. This is accomplished by the pulling action of crossbridges that are formed from the myosin filaments which attach to the actin filaments. After binding, the crossbridges shorten, thereby drawing the

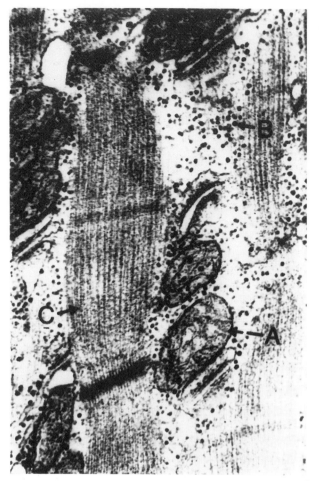

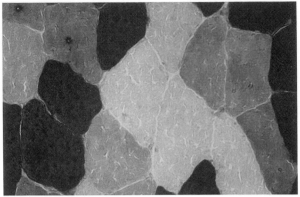

Fig. 5.3 A cross-sectional view of fibers from a human thigh muscle. The dark-stained fibers are slow twitch (ST), the lightly stained fibers are fast twitch subtype a (FTa), and the intermediately stained fibers are FTb. Courtesy of W.J. Kraemer, Pennsylvania State University.

Fig. 5.2 An electron micrograph of the interior of a muscle fiber. A = mitochondria, B = glycogen, and C = protein strands of actin and myosin (×187 500). Courtesy of D.L. Costill, Ball State University.

two protein threads past each other. In the activity of skiing, this takes place simultaneously in thousands of the muscle's fibers, resulting in force development between the attachments of the muscle on the skeleton.

Recent developments in laboratory techniques have permitted the study of the organization and function of muscles and to evaluate the effects of both training and competition on muscle. This, in turn, leads to a better understanding of the influence of training and/or conditioning on competitive performance. One characteristic of muscle fibers that has gained considerable attention in both the exercise physiology

laboratories and in the world of sport is the division of muscle cells into two groupings, the slow twitch fibers (ST) and the fast twitch fibers (FT). The FT fibers are further divided into subgroups "a" and "b." A microscopic photograph of human muscle is presented in Fig. 5.3 and the three types of fibers can be identified.

In a group of Alpine skiers, the thigh muscle will have an average of approximately 50% ST fibers, 25% FTa fibers, and 25% FTb fibers. This does not differ according to gender. However, there will be wide variation in these percentages when examining individual skiers and there is, to date, no clear indication whether it is advantageous for Alpine racers to have a greater percentage of ST or of FT fibers.

Muscle fibers function in groups called motor units and each motor unit includes only one of the three fiber types. A motor unit is comprised of a motor neuron (nerve cell) and the muscle fibers it innervates. The body of the nerve cell is located in the spinal cord where it receives its signals from other nerve cells located in the brain. An ST motor unit will include one relatively small nerve cell connected to a cluster of 10–180 muscle fibers while a FT motor unit will include a larger nerve cell which controls 300–800 muscle fibers.

ST motor units are characterized as having superior aerobic endurance and appear to be recruited most often during low-intensity endurance events such as distance running. The FTa motor units develop

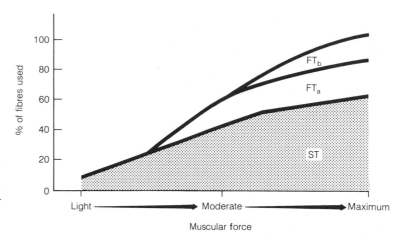

Fig. 5.4 Relationship of recruitment of the three fiber types to the force development by muscle. Light force development involves only slow twitch (ST) fibers. As force increases, fast twitch subtype a (FTa) fibers are recruited. At the highest levels of force development, all three fiber types are involved. From Costill *et al.* (1992).

considerably more force although they fatigue faster in continuous activity. For these reasons, they play an important role in short, fast events such as sprint running. Although the significance of the FTb fibers is not fully understood, it appears that these motor units are not easily recruited by the nervous system.

The pattern of recruitment among the fiber types appears to be determined principally by the athlete's requirements for force development. Figure 5.4 presents the relationship between force development by muscle and the recruitment of the motor units of the three fiber types. During low-intensity, endurance activity, almost all of the force generation is developed by ST motor units. As more force is required in the middle range of force production, FTa units contribute to an increasingly greater extent. All three motor units are involved at the highest levels of force requirement. The turns involved in Alpine racing definitely require high force development.

Studies of the fiber composition of thigh muscle (vastus lateralis) of athletes from different sport events have shown that Alpine skiers demonstrate a considerable variation but the average is a 50:50 relationship in the number of FT and ST muscle fibers. Certain élite competitors can have a 65:35 or a 35:65 relationship between the two fiber types.

This stands in direct contrast to élite cross-country skiers who can average 75% ST fibers and very few competitors will have less than a 35:65 relationship of FT to ST fibers. On the other hand, sprint runners and ice hockey players will have a higher number of FT fibers.

At this point in time, it can only be observed that no great advantage can be observed for Alpine skiers as regards predominance of one fiber type over the other when considering an athlete's potential for competitive performance. In fact, it can be stated that a more even mix of fibers is quite satisfactory and that other factors involved in the coordination of the movements and production of force and power are more important.

Muscle actions

The body contains more than 215 pairs of muscles and they vary in size, shape, and function. It is important to appreciate that every coordinated movement requires the application of force by muscles that serve as the prime movers, agonistic muscles, and the relaxation of muscles that might oppose the desired movement, the antagonistic muscles.

When the threshold of excitation of a motor unit is attained, the contractile elements of each fiber act to shorten the fiber along its longitudinal axis. Even when the fiber is prevented from shortening, the term that has been traditionally applied to this event is contraction because, without restraint, a diminishment in the length of the fiber would occur.

During the performance of sport skills, the recruitment of motor units for the purpose of developing force between the bony attachments of muscles may or may not result in the shortening of the total muscle and the drawing of the attachments closer together. Depending on the ratio between the total activation (neural signal input) to the motor units and any opposing force acting on the attachments of a muscle, the result may be either muscle shortening, muscle lengthening, or no change in the total muscle length. In forceful lengthening of the muscle, the muscle activation is not capable of causing shortening but, instead, it resists the stretch while the muscle is being lengthened.

The objective of muscle activation is to recruit selectively an appropriate pool of motor units so that the movements are controlled. The recruitment may result in shortening of the muscle, the maintenance of a particular length (as in the stabilization of body parts), or a controlled lengthening of muscle length as the distance between bony attachments increases.

To describe the active state of muscle as a "contraction" when the muscle may be shortening, maintaining the same length, or being increased in length has been determined as inappropriate. Therefore, the term muscle action has been proposed to describe the result of skeletal muscle force development interacting with the external forces that affect the body parts of an organism which, in the context of this handbook, is the Alpine skier.

Types of muscle actions

The interaction of muscle force development and the external forces will result in actions that produce static exercise (no movement about the related joints) or in dynamic exercise (involving either an increase or decrease in joint angles). Static exercise of activated muscle is traditionally referred to as isometric. Force is developed but, as there is no movement, no work is performed. All other muscle actions involve movement and are termed dynamic. The term concentric is traditionally used to identify a shortening action and the term eccentric is used to identify a lengthening action (see Table 5.2).

For the skier, the example can be given of the activity of the thigh muscles (Fig. 5.5). Starting with the skier in (a) with no upward or downward movement, the muscles exert sufficient force to maintain the position through isometric action. A controlled lowering of the body, as shown in (b), has the same muscles exerting force sufficient to regulate the speed of the lowering maneuver through eccentric action (i.e. the active muscles are forcibly stretched by gravitational pull downward as indicated by the arrows). In (c), the

Table 5.2 Classification of exercise and muscle action types

Exercise	Muscle action	Muscle length
Dynamic {	Concentric	Decreases
	Eccentric	Increases
Static	Isometric	No change

thigh muscles exert force in a concentric action to shorten themselves and bring about the elevation of the body. In a ski turn, the muscles oppose both gravity and centrifugal force by means of eccentric actions.

Isometric and dynamic actions can be assessed at any particular length of the muscle and/or positioning of the related body parts in terms of the following:
1 Directly measured force from the muscle or its tendon.
2 Force at a particular point on the related body parts.
3 Torque about the axis of rotation of each joint involved.
A dynamic action must be further described in terms of directionality (shortening or lengthening) and the velocity of muscle length change or body part movement.

Because of variation in mechanical advantage as a joint angle is changed as well as the differences in maximal force capability of a muscle through its range of length, no dynamic action of a muscle in exercise and sport performance involves constant force development. Therefore, the term isotonic is not appropriate for the description of muscle action involved in human exercise performance.

Strength and power

The ability to exert maximal force is commonly referred to as the strength of the muscles that control particular body movements. However, the muscles may perform maximal effort as either isometric, concentric, or eccentric actions and the two dynamic actions may be performed at a wide range of velocities. An infinite number of values for the strength of muscle(s) may be obtained for a human movement as

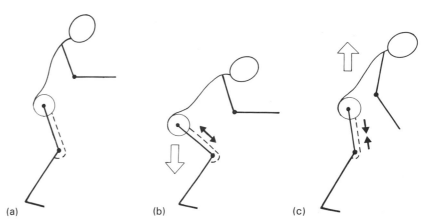

Fig. 5.5 The performance of (a) iso-metric, (b) eccentric, and (c) concentric actions by the thigh muscles of a skier.   (a)   (b)   (c)

related to the type of action, the velocity of the action, and the length of the muscle(s).

Therefore, strength is not the result of an assessment performed under a single set of conditions. Because of the number of variables or conditions involved, the strength of a muscle or muscle group can be defined as, "the maximal force generated at a specified or determined velocity" (Knuttgen & Kraemer, 1987).

For comparative purposes, the force and/or torque measurements must be performed when the muscle or muscle groups are at similar lengths or as the peak force obtained during a dynamic action. The measurements may be obtained directly from the muscle or its tendons, from a particular point on one of the body parts, or as torque developed on a testing device. Regardless of the measurement technique, the assessment must precisely identify the muscle action, the velocity of the action, and the muscle length (alternatively, the joint angle).

Power can be determined for a single body movement, a series of movements, or, as in the case of aerobic exercise, for a large number of repetitive movements. Power can be determined instantaneously at any point in a movement or averaged for any portion of a movement or bout of exercise.

For the simple movement of lifting and/or lowering a free weight, the force necessary to oppose the force of gravity acting on the free weight mass operates through a displacement (change in altitude in meters) during a determined time. Force multiplied by the displacement determines the work which, divided per unit of time, yields the power. The same determinations can be accomplished for any mechanical device where a weight stack is employed to provide the force opposing the body movement being performed.

An alternative system developed for exercise programs in rehabilitation medicine (DeLorme, 1945) has been adopted in many situations in which strength assessment and strength development is carried out. While the testing methodology does not readily yield precise information about force and/or torque development at specific muscle lengths and joint angles, the system offers the advantage of ease of test administration. Either free weights or an exercise machine can be employed.

The basic test consists of determining the number of repetitions a person can perform to exhaustion in lifting a certain mass. The mass is then described in terms of a "repetition maximum" or RM. For example, a person lifts a mass of 72 kg 10 times before exhaustion; therefore, 72 kg is identified as the person's 10 RM for the particular body movement and conditions of the test (e.g. free weight versus machine, free cadence versus controlled cadence). If the largest mass the person can lift without repetition is 98 kg, this mass is identified as the 1 RM, the person's strength score for the movement according to this procedure. Performance assessment and exercise prescription can then be accomplished in terms of the mass of a specific RM or percentages of the mass of the 1 RM. Determination of 1 RM in this manner for each body movement constitutes one approach for assessing the strength of the muscles in performing the movement.

Muscle actions in a turn

The sequence of movements in a turn involve combinations of isometric, eccentric, and concentric actions

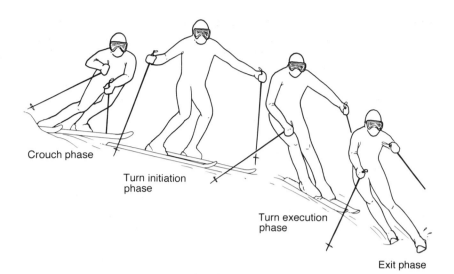

Crouch phase

Turn initiation phase

Turn execution phase

Exit phase

Fig. 5.6 Phases of a skiing turn.

of the muscles involved. This sequence is depicted in Fig. 5.6.

The skier begins in a crouch position, usually with the majority of body weight riding on the so-called downhill ski (in this case the right ski). Holding either the crouch or tuck position requires force development through isometric muscle action of the muscles (e.g. the quadriceps femoris muscles of the thigh). The skier either proceeds directly with concentric actions to produce an upward movement of the body's center of mass or engages in a slight unweighting through eccentric action and a downward counter-movement before proceeding to the concentric muscle actions that elevate the center of mass to initiate the turn.

Between the turn initiation and the turn execution, the skier reaches the high point in center of mass elevation at approximately the same time that a body rotation (with the right shoulder moving forward) produces the torsion movement resulting in the skis being transferred to a position pointing downward on the mountain (i.e. along the fall line). At this point, the skier begins shifting body weight to the left ski.

The final movements place the body weight predominantly or totally on the left ski and a controlled lowering of the body's center of mass is brought about through eccentric muscle actions. The tightness of the turn dictates the degree of torsion and the forces required by the eccentric actions. The tighter the turn, the greater is the amount of torsion and muscle force requirement. A tighter turn also involves a greater

friction between ski and snow surface which results in greater opposition to forward speed.

The large emphasis on the eccentric actions in performing the turns in Alpine skiing provides the explanation why the poorly conditioned competitor can experience muscle soreness when beginning a serious training program. This is the same soreness experienced by the recreational skier at the beginning of a skiing season. Most, if not all, of this delayed onset muscle soreness (which begins approximately 8–12 h after such exercise) is assumed to come from the microscopic injuries which occur to muscle cells not conditioned for eccentric activity.

Comparing Alpine skiing to other sport events, the demands for high force and power from the muscles is very high. Therefore, the conditioning program must include a large amount of high-resistance (or strength) training, especially during the off-season when the competitor has the time to devote to muscle development.

Energy for muscle activity

When the muscle fibers of the motor units are activated, they require energy to produce the concentric, isometric, and eccentric actions. That energy is obtained from the foods we eat in the form of carbohydrates, fats, and proteins. When broken down by digestion, these fuels yield low levels of energy that are inadequate for the immediate needs of the muscle fibers but, instead, contribute to the energy that maintains sufficient concentrations of a high-energy compound, adenosine triphosphate (ATP), that serves as the body's immediate source of energy for muscle actions as well as a wide variety of other body functions.

The muscles have four possible sources of ATP.
1 Stored within the muscle fibers.
2 Generated from energy obtained from another phosphate compound, creatine phosphate (CP).
3 Generated from energy obtained from the breakdown of carbohydrate stored in the muscle fibers as glycogen (anaerobic).
4 Generated energy obtained from the breakdown of carbohydrate and fat through oxidative metabolism (aerobic).

ATP is the immediate and only source of energy for muscle fiber activity. When it is not available to the contractile elements of the fiber, the fiber cannot continue. When a sufficient number of fibers in a muscle cannot continue, the force capability of a muscle is diminished. If the force capability is reduced to a great extent, the function of the muscle is lost and, if a sufficient percentage of the skier's musculature is unavailable, exhaustion is experienced.

CP is present within the muscle fibers and serves as a ready source of energy for the resynthesis of utilized ATP. Unfortunately the amounts of both ATP and CP in muscle are very small and, during highly intense activity such as in Alpine racing, the two compounds can only provide energy for some muscles for a short time (e.g. 5–20 s). The relationship of ATP and CP to the energy needs of muscle activity is presented in Figs 5.7 and 5.8.

During intense muscle activity, the body is not capable of providing sufficient oxygen to the fibers to regenerate sufficient ATP and the muscle fibers employ the anaerobic process of glycolysis. This involves the breakdown of the stored carbohydrate, glycogen, which results in the production of both energy and lactic acid. This process is rather inefficient and can only be utilized for short periods of time. Aerobic metabolism is 13 times more successful in yielding energy for ATP resynthesis but, as Alpine ski racing involves runs lasting 40–120 s, aerobic metabolism cannot be counted on for a major provision of energy.

During Alpine racing or intense recreational skiing, the demands on the glycolytic system are high and cause muscle lactic acid levels to rise from resting values of approximately 1 mmol/kg to over 25 mmol/

Fig. 5.7 The chemical structure of adenosine triphosphate (ATP). The diamond-shaped symbols connecting the four components indicate energy. From Maglischo (1990).

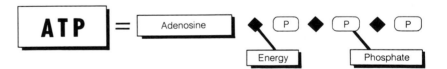

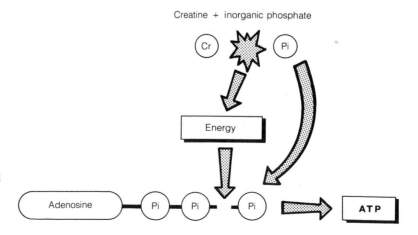

Fig. 5.8 The breakdown of creatine (Cr) and phosphate (Pi) to maintain the supply of adenosine triphosphate (ATP). From Costill *et al.* (1992).

kg of muscle. Such a high acid content in the muscle fibers inhibits further breakdown of glycogen and may also interfere with the muscle's contractile processes. Extended reliance on glycolysis (e.g. for over 2 min) for energy will result in fatigue and eventual exhaustion as the internal environment of the muscle fibers become too acidic.

Aerobic metabolism requires the availability of oxygen to the muscle fibers for the breakdown of both carbohydrate (in the form of glucose) and fat (in the form of fatty acids) in the fiber's mitochondria, structures which serve this function. Significant amounts of ATP can be resynthesized in this way but only for low to moderate intensity exercise, as in the so-called endurance events. There is a contribution of this process to the energy demands of Alpine skiing, but the skier is relying more on the contributions of CP and glycolysis.

Conditioning of muscle

There is ample evidence in the research literature that muscle tissue responds to conditioning programs through adaptations in structure and/or function. The adaptations are specific to the conditioning program as exemplified by the hypertrophy (increase in size) of FT motor units in high-resistance (or strength) programs and the increase in aerobic (oxidative) capacity of ST fibers, without change in size, to endurance training. There is still some debate concerning the possibility of conversion of motor units, ST to FT and FT to ST, in response to highly specific training programs conducted over many months. At this point in time, it can be held that, if such changes can occur, the changes in the percentage of fiber types within a particular muscle would be relatively small.

Most studies have reported that the fiber type composition of muscle appears to be fixed and not affected by training. This would mean that this aspect of potential for sports performance has been inherited. Studies with identical twins (i.e. from the same egg) have shown that they have virtually identical fiber type populations in the various muscles of their bodies whereas fraternal twins (i.e. from separate eggs) differ in fiber profiles as well as in other physical characteristics. This would support the contention that an athlete's fiber composition is determined by genetics, with the percentage of ST and FT fibers being

established soon after birth and remaining relatively unchanged throughout life.

There is good evidence, however, that transition may occur in response to specific conditioning between subgroups FTa and FTb. The FTa motor units are generally described as being more aerobic than FTb fibers and, therefore, capable of greater oxidative metabolism. With endurance conditioning, FTb motor units take on the characteristics of FTa motor units while, with high-intensity anaerobic conditioning and strength conditioning, FTa become more like FTb motor units (i.e. less aerobic and more glycolytic).

Another consideration is that the various muscles of the body demonstrate striking differences in percentages of the component fiber types within one skier. Generally, the muscles of the arms and legs have similar fiber compositions although a good example of a marked difference in each skier is between the gastrocnemius muscle (high in FT fibers) and the soleus muscle (high in ST fibers) of the calf musculature. It should also be pointed out that ST fibers are generally much larger than FT fibers and, for both fiber types, all fibers are larger in male than in female athletes.

Aerobic and anaerobic conditioning for muscle

Conditioning involves the planning and conduct of programs of exercise and nutrition which lead to adaptations of the body tissues and organs leading to improved performance for the particular sport activity. The major tissue of consideration is the skeletal muscle tissue that produces the force and power necessary to control the body movements. At one extreme of the metabolic continuum for muscle cells is the completely aerobic activity of long-distance cross-country skiing. At the other extreme are the predominantly anaerobic activities of weight lifting and short-distance sprinting. Alpine skiing is more anaerobic than aerobic although the longer the event in distance and time (as in the downhill event), the greater the contribution of aerobic metabolism to the total demand for energy.

Alpine skiing is an event involving repeated muscle actions involving high force development. Therefore, strength training and repeated bouts of anaerobic activity will result both in the increase in muscle fiber cross-sectional size (and larger musculature), increase in force production proficiency, and increases in capability of anaerobic energy release (metabolism). Proper prescription of exercise in the form of interval training can result in a simultaneous enhancement of the muscle cells' ability for aerobic metabolism.

Respiration and circulation

The muscle fibers are responsible for producing the forces for skiing performance and the energy metabolism for this force production takes place within the fibers of the recruited motor units. The muscle fibers are dependent, however, on the respiratory and circulatory systems of the body for the delivery of both energy-yielding compounds and oxygen as well as the removal of waste products during activity and recovery.

The blood carries oxygen, glucose, fatty acids, and other essential substances to capillaries in all of the body tissues. At the same time that delivery is made, the blood takes up carbon dioxide, lactic acid, and other by-products of metabolism into these same capillaries for elimination in other parts of the body. Upon return to the heart from the peripheral vessels, blood is pumped to the lungs where carbon dioxide is removed and oxygen is taken up.

At rest, heart rate (HR) may vary between 50 and 80 beats/min for the well-conditioned Alpine skier.

Generally, a low resting HR is an indication of a state of high aerobic conditioning although it does not present a precise indication of such fitness. Another factor that impacts on HR is the cluster of psychological stresses which include anticipation and anxiety. Thus, a skier at the start of a difficult run, particularly under race conditions, can be expected to have a high HR even though the "activity" of standing is not that different from lying in bedrest.

During long-lasting, aerobic endurance exercise, the HR reflects rather accurately the rate of oxygen delivery and carbon dioxide removal in proportion to the maximal rates of which the individual is capable. The point has already been made, however, that Alpine ski racing is much more of an anaerobic than aerobic event and, therefore, HR will present little insight into the intensity of the exercise other than to confirm that it rates high on scales of force and power (Fig. 5.9).

The heart of every adolescent or young adult skier will have a maximal rate which will usually run between 185 and 205 beats/min.

The amount of blood which is pumped out by the heart with each beat is termed the stroke volume (SV). A normal range of values for SV at rest for an adult is between 60 and 100 ml/beat. During intense exercise, the SV of the heart may increase 2−3 times resting values. As one might expect, the SV for aerobic endur-

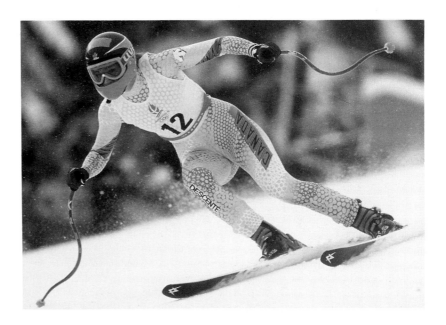

Fig. 5.9 Élite Alpine ski racers utilize strength and power, anaerobic and aerobic energy release. © Vandystadt.

ance athletes is larger both at rest and during competition than for the total population and for other
athletes. This presents the rationale for the low resting
HR for such an individual at the same time as it ex-
plains the capability for high maximal cardiac outputs
(CO in ml/min), which is determined by the product of
HR and SV. Such an athlete can supply the muscles
and other tissues of the body with more blood per
minute during competition. While high aerobic conditioning would not necessarily act to the detriment of
an Alpine skier, it is definitely not the dominant factor
in conditioning for either serious recreational skiing
or élite competition.

Respiration is the total series of processes by which
oxygen is provided to the body tissues and carbon
dioxide is removed. Respiration also plays a role in
maintenance of body fluid acid–base balance. External respiration involves the exchange of oxygen
and carbon dioxide between the lung alveoli and the
pulmonary capillaries. Internal respiration involves
the exchange of oxygen and carbon dioxide between
the capillaries of the tissues and the tissue fluids
which surround the tissue cells, such as the muscle
fibers.

Breathing, or the repetitive cycle of movement of
atmospheric air into and out of the lungs (inspiration
and expiration), serves to refresh the air that is contained in the alveoli. At rest, approximately 5 l of air
are breathed in and out each minute. During exercise,
this value is raised to over 100 l/min. Breathing is
accomplished by the skeletal muscles of the thorax,
which include the dome-shaped diaphragm muscle.
The regulation of breathing is accomplished subcon-
sciously by centers in the brain; the Alpine skier need
not be concerned about special conditioning of the
associated muscles nor in breathing appropriate to
the intensity of the exercise. Rather, the rhythm of
breathing should occur in synchrony with the performance of turning. Breathing and respiration will be
affected by lowered partial pressure of oxygen in
atmospheric air, such as at high altitude, and can be of
concern to those skiers who are predisposed to acute
mountain sickness and the related pathologies.

Oxygen uptake and $\dot{V}_{O_2 \, max}$

Oxygen uptake is assessed by measuring the rate of
oxygen that is transferred from the lungs to the blood

in the capillaries of the pulmonary circuit of the circulatory system. At rest and during light to moderate
exercise, the oxygen taken up by the blood in the
lungs becomes equivalent to the oxygen being taken
up and utilized by the cells of the peripheral tissues,
principally the skeletal muscle.

The greatest amount of oxygen uptake of which a
person is capable is referred to interchangeably as
maximal oxygen uptake, the shorthand designation of
"$\dot{V}_{O_2 \, max}$," or maximal aerobic power. This is determined by having the athlete exercise to exhaustion in
approximately 4–10 min in a so-called large muscle
activity such as running, rowing, or cross-country
skiing.

At a particular intensity of exercise, the need for
oxygen is determined by the active skeletal muscle
tissue. If the power requirement of the exercise is great
and a large number of muscle motor units are well-
conditioned for aerobic metabolism, the demand for
oxygen delivery could be great. The ability of the
delivery system relates to the capacity for cardiac
output (i.e. maximal stroke volume), the oxygen carrying capacity of the blood, the blood volume, and the
capillarization of the skeletal muscle tissue.

Élite Alpine skiers typically demonstrate
intermediate capacities for aerobic metabolism and
the criterion $\dot{V}_{O_2 \, max}$ when compared to other athlete
groups. The $\dot{V}_{O_2 \, max}$ criterion is presented as the milli-
liters of oxygen that can be delivered per kilogram
of the athlete's body mass per minute (ml/kg/min). For
example, male marathon runners and cross-country
skiers can average over 80 ml/kg, sprinters 55 ml/kg,
and Alpine skiers 65 ml/kg. From the standpoint of
capability for aerobic metabolism, the value for
Alpine skiers is quite respectable but it also indicates
that aerobic power is not of the same importance as for
the so-called endurance events. This is not surprising
when one recalls that Alpine ski races are of relatively
short duration from 40 s (slalom) up to 115 s (downhill).

The best approaches to the development of aerobic
power capabilities appropriate to the demand of
Alpine ski racing are probably best accomplished by
repeated, short-term sprint activities (e.g. 15–60 s)
that emphasize development of anaerobic capabilities at the same time that the aerobic metabolism of
the muscle cells and the oxygen delivery system are
being challenged. This type of activity together with

strength training should constitute the best preparation of muscle tissue and circulatory system for Alpine ski racing.

Fatigue and exhaustion

The term "fatigue" can be used to indicate the general sensation of tiredness as well as a decrement in performance. "Exhaustion" can be used to refer to the state when a physical activity can no longer be continued. There appear to be a number of factors in fatigue and exhaustion as related to competitive sport performance. The most commonly accepted factors in such fatigue are as follows:

1 Depletion of the energy-yielding compounds, ATP and CP.
2 Depletion of the carbohydrate stored in muscle (glycogen).
3 The accumulation in muscle of waste products, lactic acid in particular.
4 Changes in the physiochemical state of the muscle, e.g. change in mineral concentration.
5 Disturbances in the process of control of muscular activity and coordination, i.e. disturbance to central nervous system function.

As previously discussed, ATP is the immediate and only source of energy for the muscle cells and, therefore, for sports performance. CP serves as a source of energy for rapid replenishment of ATP but both compounds exist in short supply and will not permit muscle to continue to function beyond 10–30 s of high-intensity sports performance.

Both ATP and CP depend on anaerobic and aerobic mechanisms to permit the continuation of muscular activity. As previously mentioned, Alpine skiing consists of periods of activity of short duration that aerobic metabolism cannot be counted on for a very large contribution to the muscular activity involved.

The short duration of an Alpine race cannot result in the depletion of glycogen from the muscle fibers and, therefore, this cannot be a factor in fatigue. A full day of training or recreational skiing can reduce muscle glycogen levels significantly.

The association of lactic acid accumulation and fatigue has been recognized for some time. When muscle force and power development depend on anaerobic glycolysis for an extended time, large amounts of lactic acid accumulate in the active muscle fibers, particularly the FT fibers that do not have capabilities for aerobic metabolism. The accompanying accumulation of hydrogen ions which are derived from lactic acid dissociation results in a lowering of the pH (or acidosis) in the muscles. If the pH values of muscle which, at rest, average 7.1 fall as low as 6.4 because of lactic acid accumulation and dissociation, the muscles cannot continue activity and exhaustion occurs. Obviously, values between 7.1 and 6.4 in muscle can result in the lowered performance associated with the feeling of fatigue.

References

Costill, D.L., Maglischo, E.W. & Richardson, A.B. (1992) *Swimming*. Oxford: Blackwell Scientific Publications.

DeLorme, T.L. (1945) Restoration of muscle power by heavy resistance exercises. *J. Bone Joint Surg.* **27**:645–667.

Knuttgen, H.G. & Kraemer, W.J. (1987) Terminology and measurement in exercise performance. *J. Appl. Sport Sci. Res.* **1**:1–10.

Maglischo, E. (1990) *Swimming Faster*. Palo Alto, California: Mayfield Publishing.

Recommended reading

Komi, P.V. (ed.) (1992) *Strength and Power in Sport*. Oxford: Blackwell Scientific Publications.

Shephard, R.J. & Åstrand, P.-O. (eds) (1992) *Endurance in Sport*. Oxford: Blackwell Scientific Publications.

Chapter 6

Nutrition

The energy for the metabolic demands of muscular activity (force development) depends ultimately on the availability of a combination of carbohydrate and fat. During the intense activity of 0.5–2 min that an Alpine skier spends on a race course, however, the active muscles turn predominantly to the carbohydrate that is already stored in the muscle fibers. Adequate storage of carbohydrate in the body is also an important factor in supporting the vigorous activity of a skier's training program.

Carbohydrate

While the proper balance of protein, fat, vitamins, minerals, and water are essential considerations in proper nutrition, carbohydrate can be considered to be the most important nutrient for the exercising muscles of the Alpine skier. Essential for any form of athletic performance, the principal functions of carbohydrate are as follows.
1 To serve as a primary energy source for the active muscles.
2 To serve as the only source of energy for the nervous system.
3 To aid the body to use fat more effectively.

For very long-lasting endurance sports (e.g. 2 h and longer), the availability of a large supply of carbohydrate for exercise is somewhat limited by the athlete's ability to store it in the form of glycogen in the skeletal muscle fibers as well as in the liver. While a competitive ski run is completed in between 0.5 and 2 min and the Alpine skier uses but a small portion of the total glycogen storage during this short time, the skier requires a significant glycogen store for the intensive training program leading up to a competitive event. Also, the initial concentration of glycogen in the muscles is important for optimal performance in a

race. Therefore, the total storage is important from this standpoint as well.

Most athletes who follow an appropriate training diet can store approximately 1600–1800 g of glycogen. As the principal energy source for high-intensity activity, sports nutritionists advise athletes to consume diets high in carbohydrate in order to maximize their glycogen-storing potential.

High-carbohydrate diets have been recommended to athletes for a number of years. Consumption of 65–70% of total daily calories in the form of carbohydrate is the current recommendation. However, surveys of athletes concerning their dietary patterns reveal that their total carbohydrate intake is closer to 45–50% of total caloric intake. This discrepancy is somewhat alarming in light of the negative impact that a low-carbohydrate diet can have on glycogen storage and, therefore, on performance both in training and in competition.

A careful examination of a skier's knowledge of carbohydrate sources can help reveal where dietary shortfalls occur. The following list of food sources high in carbohydrate may be useful as a guide to evaluating or planning carbohydrate consumption (Table 6.1).

How much carbohydrate should Alpine skiers consume?

Diets comprised of at least 65% carbohydrate are best for athletes who have increased energy demands. The typical competitive athlete requires at least 3000 kcal (Calories) per day to sustain normal body function (and body weight) and much more if the exercise training program is intense or prolonged. This translates to a minimum of 2000 kcal from carbohydrate or 500 g (for carbohydrate, there are 4 kcal/g). The larger the athlete, the larger the total caloric demand, but the 65% rule will always pertain.

When selecting foods for breakfast, lunch, dinner, or snacks, athletes should constantly strive to choose foods that improve the carbohydrate profile. A useful formula for increasing carbohydrates in each meal is to include the following.
1 One to two pieces of fruit.
2 One to two cups of low-fat milk, 56–84 g (2–3 oz) low-fat cheese, or 224 g (8 oz) of yogurt.

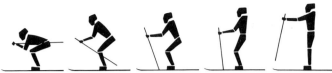

Table 6.1 Typical sources of carbohydrate (CHO) for the skier

Carbohydrate sources	CHO (g)	Total kcal	CHO (%)	Protein (%)	Fat (%)
Bread (2 slices)	25	132	76	13	11
Bagel (1)	31	163	76	16	8
Pasta (1 cup)	44	216	81	13	6
Rice (1 cup)	50	223	90	8	2
Potato (med. baked)	21	95	88	10	2
Muffin (med. blueberry)	19	126	61	8	31
English muffin (1)	26	135	77	13	10
Pancakes (3 med.)	42	210	80	13	7
Waffle (1 large)	36	285	50	7	43
French toast (2)	34	306	44	15	41
Banana (1 med.)	27	108	99	0.5	0.5
Apple (1 med.)	20	80	100	0	0
Orange (1 med.)	16	65	99	0.8	0.2
Pear (1 med.)	25	100	100	0	0
Yams (1 med.)	38	158	96	4	0
Corn on the cob (small)	21	100	84	13	3
Carrots (2/3 cup)	7	31	90	10	0
Peas (1/2 cup)	11	62	71	29	0
Vegetable juice (1 cup)	11	37	90	9	1

3 Three to five servings from the grain group (bread, cereal, pasta, rice, etc.).
4 One to two servings of vegetables.

Timing of carbohydrate ingestion

A common misconception regarding sports nutrition for performance is that of attaching too much importance to the content of the meals taken just prior to exercise or competition. In reality, nutritional practices during the entire course of a training program leading up to a competitive event have the greatest impact on how an athlete will perform on the race day. If an athlete typically eats a low-carbohydrate diet, training performance will likely be sub-optimal and this will ultimately influence overall competitive status. Therefore, the athlete should concentrate nutritional efforts on the diet program during the training period and simply continue to apply those principles to the pre- and post-competition dietary regimens. At all times, the basic consideration for all meals is high carbohydrate content.

The pre-competition meal

Many athletes have idiosyncratic eating behaviors prior to competition. They believe that a particular food or eating plan will promote winning. Although an athlete may perform satisfactorily after eating a donut and drinking a carbonated beverage, the risk of compromising a better performance that could have been obtained from superior "fuel" may not be worth it.

Most sports nutritionists recommend a pre-competition meal that occurs 3–4 h prior to the event, since digestion requires this much time. The meal should still consist of at least 65% carbohydrate along with a low fiber content. The rationale for a high-carbohydrate pre-competition diet is based on how nutrients empty from the stomach. Carbohydrates empty first, protein second, and fat last. Due to this emptying order, the pre-competition diet should be relatively low in fat, allowing the athlete to perform with an empty stomach. Total intake should not exceed 500–600 kcal. Foods to consider as good pre-competition carbohydrate sources include: low-fiber cereals, non-fat milk or yogurt, fruit juices, low fiber fruits (e.g. bananas, oranges), pasta and sauce, low-fiber breads with jam, jelly, or honey.

Post-competition meals

Carbohydrate replacement after a race is essential, primarily to replace glycogen stores. When muscle glycogen is depleted, the athlete experiences fatigue and a sense of tiredness. Mistakes and injuries thus occur more frequently. Consuming carbohydrate-rich foods soon after training or a race (within 2 h) is optimal for glycogen resynthesis. It takes approximately 24 h to replace glycogen stores completely, which has importance for those athletes competing in intensive daily training.

Protein

Alpine skiers require between 0.8 and 1 g of protein per kilogram of body weight per day (the recommended dietary allowance or RDA). This standard applies to both female and male skiers. Although the misconception of greater protein needs for muscle hypertrophy still exists, research has demonstrated that only those athletes who compete in ultra-endurance events, such as marathons or ultra-marathons, full triathlons, and endurance cycling events, require a slightly higher consumption of protein. Even then, the maximum amount of protein suggested is 1.2–1.6 g/kg/day. This amount is typically found in the diets of most athletes without their paying any special attention to the issue.

One can frequently read in food advertisements that athletes require much greater amounts of protein if one goal of the conditioning program is increased strength (as related to muscle hypertrophy). This logic has proven to be an effective marketing gimmick but, physiologically, is quite simply without basis. To increase lean tissue, the athlete must increase total calories in conjunction with the initiation of a serious strength training regimen. Daily caloric composition should consist of the standard dietary rules: 65–70% carbohydrate, 12–15% protein, and less than 30% fat.

Foods high in protein include both animal and plant sources. One benefit from obtaining protein from meat is the addition of the mineral, iron. A benefit from milk-based protein is the addition of the mineral, calcium. Both minerals are thought to be underconsumed in many female athlete's diets.

Two other misconceptions surrounding protein exist. The first is that of protein quality. Many coaches and trainers think that protein from plant sources is of such a low quality that it is not useful for providing necessary amino acids. The truth is that plant proteins actually do not contain all the essential amino acids, so they must be combined (two or more sources consumed at a meal). When the plant sources are combined, such as beans and rice or bread and peanut butter, the mix of amino acids becomes complete and the protein is just as useful as amino acids from animal protein. An important consideration is that all vegetables and grains (in other words all plants) contain amino acids in varying amounts. Typically, the amino acids missing in plants can be easily combined, therefore simply eating two or more plant foods each day is the key to complementing proteins.

Some examples of complementing protein sources include: beans with rice; bread with any vegetable; seeds with wheat products; and corn with any other vegetable.

In addition, eating one plant source of protein with an animal source automatically makes the amino acids in the plant useful for forming new body proteins.

The second misconception concerns that of the amount of protein found in meats other than red meat. All animal-based proteins contain the full complement of amino acids. Therefore, any animal food or meat is a high-quality protein. Eggs and milk are the two most biologically available forms of protein. Both can be eaten relatively fat-free by discarding the egg yolk and choosing skimmed milk.

Fat

A low fat diet is the recommendation made by most nutritionists, even for those athletes trying to gain weight. Although fat is an essential nutrient, the amount in the diet should not exceed 30% of total calories. As a matter of fact, many athletes are already successfully consuming diets consisting of 20% fat. Fats to focus on when choosing fat sources are mono-unsaturated fats, such as olive, peanut, and canola oils. Polyunsaturated fats, such as corn, soy, cottonseed, and sunflower seed oils are better than saturated fats. The saturated fats to avoid are butter, palm oil, and coconut oil.

As diets become increasingly higher in carbohydrates, they typically become lower in fat. If undesirable weight loss should occur, the answer is simply to increase total calories while keeping the proportion of carbohydrates within the range of 65–70%. A carbohydrate-rich beverage (shake drink) will help boost needed calories lost due to a lower fat regime.

The goal of a low fat diet is to avoid added fat (such as frequently found in dressings, gravy, sauces, and spreads) while continuing to eat nutrient-rich foods that may contain fat, such as lean meats and low fat cheeses.

Iron

Supplementing a diet with minerals and vitamins is still a controversial subject when it applies to athletes. Typically, an athlete can obtain all of the necessary nutrients from selecting a variety of foods from the fruit, vegetable, grain, milk, and meat groups. One major exception to this thought, however, is that of iron for female athletes. Some research has shown that, in order for a woman to obtain the RDA for iron, she needs to consume at least 2000 kcal daily from a variety of food sources. Food intake surveys from female athletes have revealed that many do consume this number of calories. In addition, the food choices female athletes make have a tendency to be lower in the meat category as they attempt to limit their fat intake.

Vegetarian athletes should be made aware of plant sources of iron, such as dried beans, which provide the best source. An iron supplement may be indicated for some female and vegetarian athletes.

The anti-oxidant nutrients – vitamins C and E, beta-carotene, and selenium

Several studies have demonstrated that free radical production (chemicals produced in the body that have unpaired electrons) is increased in both competitive athletes and strenuous exercisers. As free radicals increase, there is increased tissue damage. Vitamins C and E, beta-carotene (the vitamin A precursor), and selenium are thought to be free radical scavengers. In other words, these nutrients have shown efficacy in

reducing free radical production by protecting cell membranes. As a result, they are linked with aiding the prevention of heart disease, certain cancers, cataracts, and the aging process.

Studies have not clearly determined whether the anti-oxidant nutrients should be increased in the diets of persons engaged in vigorous exercise programs, although it is clear that free radical production is greater in strenuous exercisers. The best recommendation to date is to increase those foods that contain the anti-oxidant nutrients. The best sources of vitamin C are citrus fruits and juices, broccoli, potatoes, tomatoes, cabbage, green peppers, and berries. The best sources of beta-carotene are orange-colored vegetables such as carrots, yams, sweet potatoes, and squash. High beta-carotene fruits include apricots, peaches, nectarines, and cantaloupe. Vitamin E rich foods are vegetable oils including nuts and seeds. Lastly, foods rich in selenium include seafood and liver. Meat in general provides the next best source of this element.

Liquid supplements

Most athletes are able to obtain the necessary macronutrients (carbohydrate, protein, and fat) and micronutrients (vitamins and minerals) from normal foods found in any grocery store. The notion that a specially formulated sports supplement will offer a greater performance edge has not been established and the commercial products are typically overpriced for their basic contents. Unfortunately, athletes have a high predisposition for believing that liquid carbohydrate or protein supplements will promote peak performance. The reality is that both liquid supplements and foods offer nutrients and energy which are key to optimal performance.

The real question for coaches and trainers to consider is whether athletes need special products. In most cases, sports nutritionists will hold that regular food supplies everything the athlete needs. Exceptions to this rule include the following:
1 If weight is not being successfully maintained and the athlete is already consuming appropriate meals and snacks, a liquid supplement is an easier way to increase calories without making the athlete feel overly full and uncomfortable.
2 If weight gain is desired and the athlete is already consuming a large number of calories from good food

sources, liquid supplements are easy to drink between meals.

3 For pre- or post-competition meals, liquid carbohydrate supplements have been shown to be easily digested while not leaving an athlete feeling full. Protein supplements are discouraged with skiers since a reasonable diet with varied foods should be expected to provide adequate protein.

Fluids

Hydration is one of the most important determinants of how well an athlete will perform, whether on a training or competition day. With the advent of new sports drinks coming onto the market at record rates, many athletes, coaches, and trainers are beginning to question the role and purpose of these products as opposed to water. Initially, the purpose of sports drinks was to replenish minerals lost in sweat, particularly certain electrolytes: sodium, potassium, and chloride. Today, we know that these elements are lost in microscopic amounts, even in the most strenuous exercisers. What is lost can easily be replaced by eating a normal diet after exercise. For skiers, this is certainly the case. Athletes who exercise in hot climates for very long periods of time are the ones who must be alert to excessive sweat loss.

Many studies have evaluated the efficacy of carbohydrate/electrolyte sports beverages to determine whether they do indeed enhance performance. In studies of cyclists, carbohydrate beverage users outperformed water users by several seconds. In other studies, carbohydrate beverages appear to be the preferred drink, both during and after competition. Athletes claim that the taste is better than water and,

therefore, they have a greater likelihood for rehydrating.

Water is as perfectly useful as a special hydration and rehydration fluid. Skiers should be encouraged to drink more water throughout the entire day as opposed to only prior to or after an exercise session. Water can be flavored with lemon or lime to enhance its flavor if taste will help the skier to maintain appropriate hydration.

Skiers should not require additional carbohydrate from a sports drink during competition. However, on a training day after skiing several hours, a sports beverage can provide an easily digestible form of carbohydrate in addition to maintaining hydration.

Altitude and appetite suppression

There is good evidence that some persons experience a loss of appetite when moving to altitude. This can be related to thyroid suppression and acid–base balance change that can last for a few days. While this phenomenon is quite common for persons engaging in exercise at very high altitudes, such as in mountain climbing, it can occur in skiers training and competing at so-called "intermediate altitudes." Difficulty in sleeping can also occur and the resultant feeling of fatigue can contribute to a lack of interest in food.

It is most often a transient experience for skiers and should not be of any great concern to competitive skiers who spend long periods of time at the altitudes common to international competition sites. However, skiers should be aware of the possibility of the phenomenon and take it into consideration when planning menus and maintaining appropriate body weight.

Chapter 7

Training

The physical requirements for Alpine skiing differ when a comparison is made between the recreational skier and the ski racer. Although these differences are relatively small, they can influence the choice of pre- and in-season conditioning programs. There is nothing magic about training for Alpine skiing. The most successful skiers over the last few years have relied on exercises which are relatively simple yet specific for the rigors of their sport.

A recent study done through the Sports Medicine Council of the United States Ski Team has quantified the training requirements for Alpine skiing and compared the physiologic needs of the recreational skier to the competitive skier. In addition, a separate study has shown a relationship between specific training parameters and competitive performance.

The specific requirements include muscle endur- ance, strength, power, plus both aerobic and anaerobic conditioning. Another requirement for skiing which is not necessary to the same extent in other sports is the need for repetitive concentric and eccentric qua- driceps contractions without a rest period. Ski train- ing techniques may change, but the physical par- ameters remain constant.

The most important muscle group to be targeted is the quadriceps. This is the major muscle group that maintains the skier's position in space, defining the delicate balance required for executing a turn. As this muscle fatigues, the delicate balance is altered, creat- ing a potential inability to recover from a fall. This makes the skier more susceptible to injury and inter- feres with performance. While the quadriceps is the key muscle to condition, it does not function inde- pendently. The quadriceps/hamstring relationship is particularly important and its effectiveness can be maintained with weight-bearing and closed kinetic chain exercise. The agonist—antagonist relationship of all muscles up and down the kinetic chain makes the use of functional exercise helpful in developing the strength, power, and endurance necessary for Alpine skiing. Training which isolates the agonist without including the antagonist (quadriceps while ignoring the hamstring) can be useful if specific areas of weak- ness are identified, but it is usually possible to exer- cise both simultaneously in weight-bearing exercise

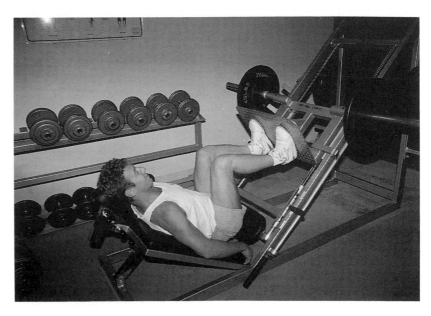

Fig. 7.1 Leg press.

which maintains the physiologic relationship between the two (Fig. 7.1).

Confidence through training

Confidence is important to the competitive skier. Eriksson noted that when skiers of different abilities were analyzed for the type of muscle fiber they used during skiing, experienced skiers used a preponderance of slow twitch and fast twitch a (STa and FTa) fibers. There was little or no reduction in glycogen in the voluntary FTb fibers. Inexperienced skiers used primarily the fast twitch or voluntary fibers, therefore, tiring much more quickly than the advanced skiers. The confidence gained from improved skiing ability seems to reduce the reliance of the skier upon the FTb fibers.

Specificity of training

It is important to realize that skiing involves not only the lower extremity. The upper and mid body participate in each turn. Ideal specificity of exercise involves activities which simulate skiing and uses muscles involved in the ski turn while supplying the aerobic and anaerobic requirements for the sport. Examples of exercise which involve the ski-specific muscles include elastic resistance training, racquet sports, uphill and downhill running, hiking, rowing ergometer, stepper devices, and soccer (Fig. 7.2). Another sport which enhances endurance, strength, and power to the quadriceps is intense cycling. However, since it permits only the concentric contraction it should be an adjunct to exercises involving both types of contraction. Flexibility is necessary during all stages of training, and its maintenance can avoid injury.

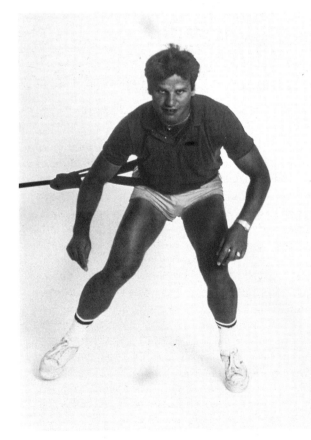

(a)

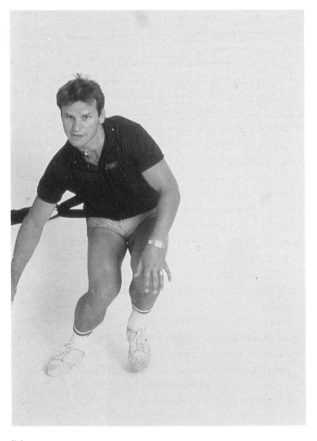

(b)

Fig. 7.2 Sport Cord side-to-side exercise. A ski-specific type of exercise that requires agility and power.

Strength

Strength is an important factor in Alpine skiing. Strength may be defined as the maximal force that can be exerted in a single voluntary contraction. It is basic to motor performance and may be the most important single factor in ski racing performance. All physical activities depend on the ability of the body and its parts to work against resistance. Strength is the basis of muscular endurance, agility, coordination, and balance. In Alpine skiing, strength in the lower extremities, upper and mid body is crucial. Balance during a ski turn is maintained by the muscles of the torso and arms, and strength in these areas can help a skier recover equilibrium.

Strengthening of the lower extremities should focus on the quadriceps as well as the muscles of the hip, foot, and ankle. Quadriceps strength can be addressed in several ways.

Isometric contractions can be used against a fixed resistance. Isometric exercise can be effective in duplicating the "thigh burn" which is present in Alpine skiing. The wall sit (using the wall as a back rest with the knees bent at 90° and staying in this position for long periods of time) can be a beneficial exercise for skiing, but care should be taken to avoid patellar pain due to the pressure placed on the patella during this exercise. If you have known patellofemoral problems avoid this exercise.

Dynamic exercise can also be used in strength training for skiing. Knee extensions represent a good concentric type of quadriceps exercise. The knee extension can, however, precipitate patellofemoral problems. These exercises should be done initially with the hand on the patella, and if crepitus exists, the knee extension exercise should be done in two parts, eliminating the mid-part of the range (60–30°) that usually precipitates crepitus. Occasionally crepitus is present in the knee as the knee reaches full extension, in which case this range should be eliminated. The knee extension exercise can be done with several types of exercise apparatus. A weight boot or ankle weight can be used for knee extensions (Fig. 7.3). One problem with the knee extension using ankle weights or a weight boot is that the lower part of the extension, from 90 to 60°, has minimal resistance, and a pendulum effect is created in this lower range. If there is crepitus in the 60–30° range and this is eliminated,

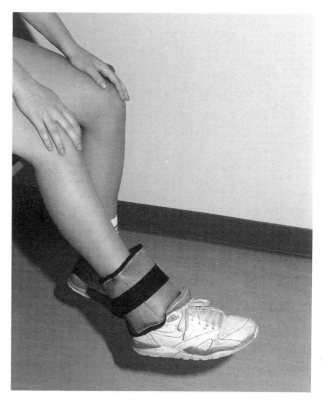

Fig. 7.3 A knee extension exercise using an ankle weight.

this limits the effective exercise to a short-arc quad from approximately 30° to full extension. If the goal is to use the 90–60° range, then exercise equipment which supplies resistance at the ankle through the full range should be used. This would include elastic exerciser and machine exercises. Dynamic equipment, variable resistance exercisers and isokinetic exercisers can all provide this type of resistance.

Generally, these exercises are done with three sets of 10 repetitions at approximately 70% of the maximum weight which can be used for one lift.

A second type of strength training device which does not incorporate specificity but only focuses on specific muscle groups is variable resistance exercise. This would include Nautilus, Eagle, Keiser, and other exercise devices which vary the resistance to match the strength changes through a range of motion. These exercise devices can be effective. However, the same concerns for patellofemoral problems and lack of specificity must be considered during their use in exercise.

A third type of exerciser which can build strength but also power and endurance is the isokinetic exercise equipment. The addition of speed as a parameter during the exercise has some benefits, and for testing, these pieces of equipment can quantify multiple factors. These exercisers are mainly nonspecific, but some incorporate an eccentric component to complement the concentric component. Examples of this type of device would be Lido, Cybex, Biodex, and Ariel exercisers. Lack of specificity would be a consideration in this type of exercise, but the ability to incorporate speed in training is appealing.

Another type of device which can be used for strength training is free weights. Free weights have several advantages as they are portable, relatively inexpensive, and provide not only strength training, but the requirement for balance and coordination during the exercise. In general, free weights would be used during early and mid-season training for Alpine skiing.

Specific areas of intensity in exercise would be the quadriceps with knee extension (taking care to avoid patellofemoral problems), hamstring curls to address the hamstring, and squats. These exercises should be done to varying degrees of depth to address strength training with a degree of specificity, using both concentric and eccentric contraction. A leg press device is also effective and specific for skiing as it involves both concentric and eccentric contraction. A wide range of upper and mid-body exercises are available to complement the lower body exercises.

Power

Power is defined as force times displacement (which equals work) divided by time. Power can be thought of as the ability to use strength in an athletic manner. This is an area which can be improved through training. Another way to view it would be force times distance divided by time. In effect, power is a way of quantifying the rate of doing work. Power is an important parameter in Alpine skiing.

The speed of exercise is important in most competitive sports. The ability to create an explosive start and to correct suddenly and change directions rapidly are elements of power. With this is mind, exercise which builds power can be divided into several types. One is a machine-type power training, utilizing equip-

ment discussed in strength training. These devices are Lido, Cybex, etc., and they allow the athlete to do strength training with a speed parameter added. This is effective as far as muscle training is concerned, but ignores muscle specificity for the specific sport.

Another approach to power training is to use the elastic resistance device as a resistance trainer, and do power training during functional exercises which are specific for the sport. The elastic resistance device has become extremely important in training techniques for Alpine skiing.

More specifically, the Sport Cord has been used by the United States Alpine Team as the basis for their power training for several years, and has been an effective exerciser, providing both power and specificity of exercise. Another power exerciser and quantifier is the Vertec (Fig. 7.4). This device quantifies the vertical leap and trains the individual to recruit more muscle fibers, thus increasing power.

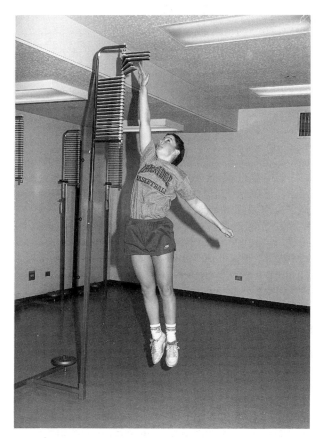

Fig. 7.4 The Vertec.

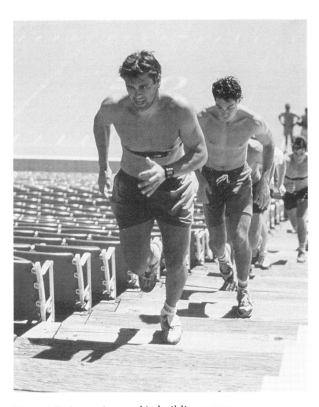

Fig. 7.5 Stair running used in building power.

Hiking, hill running, and circuit training can also build power, using the body alone as a resistance (Fig. 7.5).

An additional advantage to power training is that it enhances the ability to recover in an injury-producing situation. It is the ability to use strength quickly through time that allows these recoveries to occur. If you have watched a downhill race where a skier goes out of control and pulls back into control, it is the muscle power which provides this ability coupled with the strength necessary to provide the power.

Endurance

Endurance is particularly important in Alpine skiing, as the sport requires high intensity of exercise over a 1–2 min period. Eriksson has shown that the muscle fiber types used during this period are mostly STa and FTa fibers. This indicates that endurance training would be an extremely important addition to incorporate along with the strength and power discussed earlier. Specificity of endurance training can be used at the later stages, but initially the use of endurance training for specific muscle fiber types is important. Exercise devices which can be used for this type of training includes cycling with high intensity, rowing ergometer, hiking and jogging, and the use of elastic resistance cord. The ability to do long-term one-third squats, long-term side-to-side exercises with resistance and intensity, and running against resistance all incorporate endurance training and create the "thigh burn" necessary to build endurance. Other exercisers including the Skier's Edge may be used in specific training of muscle fiber types.

When endurance is depleted, the muscle loses its ability to provide power, thus affecting performance and ability to recover balance in Alpine skiing.

Agility

Agility is the capacity to change position and direction rapidly and precisely without loss of balance. In order to have agility, it is necessary to have built a base of strength, power, and endurance. The endurance factor is important in that as endurance decreases, power and agility is lost concomitantly. Thus, in order to build agility, it is necessary to have development of strength, power, and endurance first (Fig. 7.6).

Agility can be trained for through the use of specific exercises which simulate the sport. In ski racing, this would include sports which require strength, power, endurance, and repetitive concentric/eccentric contractions. This can be simulated with exercise devices such a Sport Cord and Skier's Edge, but can also be obtained through other sports which do not simulate skiing specifically but require the repetitive concentric/eccentric contractions and sudden changes of direction. This would include soccer, racquet sports, skating, and motorcross among others. Downhill running can also be included in this group and is very specific for Alpine ski racing, but can aggravate a patellofemoral or knee instability problem and this should be carefully considered.

Balance

Dynamic balance is the ability to maintain equilibrium during vigorous movements. This depends

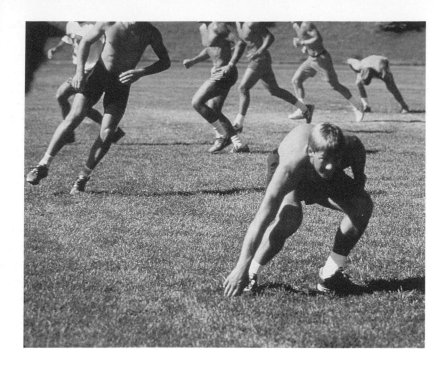

Fig. 7.6 Girardelli-type exercise used in building agility.

on the ability to integrate multiple areas of input, including visual input, muscle receptor input, and information from the semi-circular canals of the inner ear. Training for balance is extremely difficult, but this can be incorporated with exercises such as Sport Cord (Fig. 7.7). Balance exercises can be done during on-snow training, but are difficult to quantify. On-snow ski drills incorporating skiing on one ski and skiing without poles are examples of exercises which enhance balance.

Coordination

Coordination ties together all of the factors including strength, power, endurance, agility, and balance. The coordination for a specific sport is best gained through performance of that sport. Activities which closely simulate it can be used, but in the sport of skiing, skiing is the best way to build skiing coordination.

Flexibility

Use of static stretching in maintenance of flexibility can enhance performance and avoid injury. Judicious use of static stretching is encouraged throughout any muscle training program.

Amongst the muscle groups which need to maintain flexibility for the ski racer are the posterior calf mus-

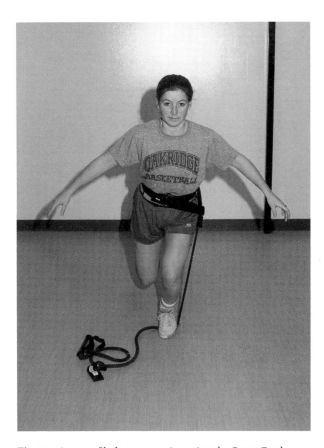

Fig. 7.7 A type of balance exercise using the Sport Cord.

cles and the Achilles tendon, the quadriceps and hamstrings, and the thigh adductors. Slow sustained stretching of these groups prior to exercise periods or skiing will help maintain the flexibility needed. For ski racers trunk flexibility is also a major factor and this should be factored into any ski racing conditioning program.

Anaerobic training

The high intensity of strength and power production involved in Alpine ski racing places great demands on the anaerobic metabolic capacities of the skeletal muscles. Anaerobic metabolism is relatively inefficient and results in the production of lactic acid. As a result of increased lactic acid production and increased carbon dioxide production, both heart rate and lung ventilation are increased.

It is important to realize that untrained individuals have a low anaerobic threshold (the point at which the requirement for anaerobic metabolism is reached) whereas, with sufficient endurance training, it is possible to elevate this threshold and increase the contribution of aerobic metabolism to the total production of energy for muscle activity. This will diminish the appearance of the byproducts of anaerobic metabolism which negatively affect athletic performance.

One method of training for anaerobic exercise is to increase the aerobic capacity of the ski racer. The use of interval training after a high aerobic capacity has been attained seems to be the most effective way of reaching this goal in Alpine skiing. The use of uphill sprints, high-intensity cycling, and interval training coupled with activities of maintenance for aerobic capacity constitutes an effective program for attaining the necessary level of conditioning. Soccer, basketball, and other sports which provide high-intensity exercise coupled with short rest periods are all helpful in providing this aerobic–anaerobic training combination.

Aerobic training

Aerobic exercise is exercise which requires oxygen for the release of energy in the active muscle cells. While fat is also utilized, the aerobic metabolism of carbohydrate is the body's most effective method of energy production for skeletal muscle activity. Although

anaerobic metabolism seems to be the major system used during Alpine ski racing, aerobic conditioning plays a major role in the total conditioning program for the skier.

Aerobic exercise results in no lactic acid production, lactic acid being an end-product of anaerobic metabolism. Lactic acid contributes to labored breathing and muscle discomfort. A welcome side-effect of aerobic exercise conditioning is its effect on stress management. The hormonal effects of exercise are being studied, but it is clear that the hormonal effect of aerobic training is beneficial.

As the intense exertion involved in an Alpine ski race commences, both the aerobic and anaerobic mechanisms of cellular metabolism are challenged to produce energy for the production of force by the muscle cells. Pulmonary ventilation is augmented and lactic acid concentrations increase in the exercising muscles as well as in rest of the body. During the course of the ski run, the better the aerobic conditioning the greater the amount of energy the muscles can derive from aerobic metabolism, thus diminishing the demand on anaerobic metabolism. Effective training for Alpine ski racing involves both aerobic and anaerobic components in the total training program. It is important, however, not to overemphasize long-duration exercise as too much aerobic conditioning can have a negative effect on strength, power, and anaerobic performance.

Tests have been conducted to define the level of aerobic conditioning involved with Alpine ski competition. Due to the use of dry land training techniques, the level of aerobic conditioning is relatively high in Alpine skiers but not comparable to long-term endurance athletes. A wide variation is observed in the maximal oxygen uptake values of élite ski racers (Fig. 7.8), confirming that very high levels of aerobic conditioning are not necessary for success. Although hereditary factors influence the capacity of an individual for aerobic performance, it is clear that any person whose goal is to be a ski racer can build the aerobic capacity necessary for Alpine ski racing.

In training for aerobic capacity, the use of long-duration exercise such as jogging, cycling, cross-country skiing, or hiking are commonly used. Soccer, basketball, and any sport that requires a large amount of intensive running coupled with short breaks are helpful in building the aerobic capacity. As aerobic

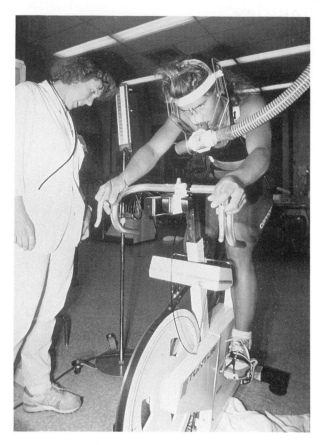

Fig. 7.8 Maximal oxygen consumption testing.

power is increased, it is possible to rely on interval training to enhance aerobic capacity. This can be accomplished with high-intensity hiking, cycling, uphill running, team sports, and other activities which require repeated bouts of high-intensity exertion.

Conclusion

In order to train for Alpine ski racing, it is important to plan training to coincide with the season. In general, strength, power, endurance, aerobic, and anaerobic training should be done during the non-skiing periods. During these times, specificity can be considered but not emphasized. During on-snow periods, maintenance exercises can be performed, but the emphasis should be on specificity, building on the base which is obtained during the off-snow period. Ideal specificity is the use of skiing for training, enhancing agility, balance, and coordination. The conditioning base should have been built prior to the on-snow training.

During the competitive season, it has been shown that conditioning levels can be decreased unless specific maintenance programs are maintained. This loss is due to the relative inactivity caused by travel, weather conditions, and "staleness" caused by too much skiing. A balance should be maintained in order to avoid overtraining during this period.

Recommended reading

Karlsson, J., Eriksson, A., Forsberg, A., Kallerg, L. & Tesch, P. (1978) *The Physiology of Alpine Skiing*. Park City, Utah: US Ski Coaches Association.

Steadman, J.R., Swanson, K.R., Atkins, J.W. & Hagerman, G.R. (1987) Training for Alpine skiing. *Clin. Orthop. Rel. Res.* **216**:34–38.

Trepp-White, A. & Johnson, S. (1991) Physiological comparison of international, national and regional skiers. *Int. J. Sports Med.* **12(4)**:374–378.

Section 3

Injuries

Chapter 8

Head

Head trauma can be anticipated in almost any type of athletic event, and nearly half the fatalities in all athletic endeavors result from trauma to the head and neck. While most Americans think about football as the primary cause of head and neck injuries in sports, winter sports, and especially Alpine skiing, cause many head injuries that encompass all known types of head trauma. Consequently, individuals at every level who are involved with skiing as well as the skiers themselves should be trained in the recognition, evaluation, and initial management of the head-injured Alpine skier. This chapter provides basic information on head injuries in Alpine skiers with special emphasis on the types of head injuries, risk factors involved, recognition and care of the head-injured patient, prevention of such injuries, and return to sport following head injury.

Mechanisms and classification of injuries

Head injuries sustained in Alpine skiing can vary from the minor, such as a scalp bruise, to the very severe in which there is actual brain tissue damage such as cerebral laceration with tearing of the brain tissue. Regardless of the severity, the mechanism of head injury is a direct result of either a static or dynamic load being applied to the head. Static loads are usually defined as those with a duration of application which exceeds 200 ms, and dynamic loads are less than 200 ms, but more frequently are in the range of 5–50 ms.

Static or slow loads as a cause of head injuries in skiers are relatively uncommon. Static load head-injured patients seldom lose consciousness. In fact, the disassociation between the severe focal injury and the maintenance of consciousness is quite remarkable.

Rapid impact to the head is much more common in skiing accidents and often results from collision with fixed objects. This dynamic impact includes both the contact phenomena as well as the inertial loading of the head and its contents. The inertial load portion of a dynamic head injury can also occur during the violent flexion–extension movements of the head after a high-speed collision of skiers. This inertial loading is a significant part of the overall injury mechanism.

Head injuries can be generally classified as either diffuse or focal. Focal injuries are usually the result of post-traumatic intracranial mass lesions and include subdural hematomas, epidural hematomas, cerebral contusions, and intracerebral hematomas. Diffuse brain injuries are also post-traumatic, but they are not directly associated with focal intracranial lesions. They usually produce more severe brain dysfunction that results from increasing amounts of acceleration damage to the brain. Diffuse brain injury which involves structural damage is the most severe type of injury because there is actual axonal disruption within the brain. Milder brain injuries such as mild concussion in which there is no structural damage are less severe because the integrity of the central nervous system elements remains intact.

Diffuse brain injuries in Alpine skiers include cerebral concussion and diffuse axonal injury. In general terms, a cerebral concussion is produced by a nonfocal brain injury which results in neurologic dysfunction. The neurologic functional impairment usually is immediate and transient in such injuries. The victim may be unconscious or remain conscious but suffer disorientation, amnesia, dizziness, or disequilibrium. More specifically, Gennarelli has emphasized that a head injury should not be defined as a concussion if the resulting unconsciousness persists for longer than 6 h. He also states that cerebral concussions produce neurologic dysfunction without substantial anatomic disruption.

Gennarelli divides cerebral concussions into mild and classic. He further segregates mild concussions into three subcategories based on their severity. These categories can be applied to most head injuries sustained by athletes including Alpine skiers. The mildest form of concussion results in confusion and disorientation without amnesia, whereas the moderate type includes retrograde amnesia (no specific memory of events which immediately preceded the injury or the injury itself). This retrograde amnesia may not develop for 5–10 min after the head injury, but it usually is permanent in spite of eventual full neurological recovery. The most severe form of mild concussion includes confusion and disorientation as well as both retrograde and posttraumatic amnesia. The retrograde and some posttraumatic amnesia may be permanent after the remainder of the dysfunction is resolved.

Classic cerebral concussion is more severe than the mild concussion described above. Classic concussion involves a full loss of consciousness as a direct result of the head injury. There is both retrograde and post-traumatic amnesia associated with classic concussion. The duration of the unconsciousness, which occurs at the moment of impact, is directly related to the severity of the head trauma. If the unconsciousness exceeds 6 h, diffuse axonal injury may be present. Brain contusions and skull fractures are also frequently seen with the classic cerebral concussion.

When post-traumatic unconsciousness or coma exceeds 6 h in duration, the likely etiology is a diffuse brain injury with axonal disruption. Gennarelli has classified diffuse axonal injuries into the distinct categories of mild, moderate, and severe based on the severity and duration of the coma. Unconsciousness usually persists for 6–24 h with the mildest form of diffuse axonal injury. There is usually mild to moderate memory deficit but usually no motor deficit. The post-traumatic amnesia may persist for several hours.

The most common type of diffuse axonal injury as defined by Gennarelli is the moderate form. The ensuing unconsciousness usually lasts for more than 24 h but lacks any prominent or permanent brain stem signs. This type of injury usually is associated with basal skull fractures. The retrograde and post-traumatic amnesia may persist for long periods, and often there are permanent deficits of intellectual, memory, and personality functions which may be mild to severe.

The severe diffuse axonal injury is the most devastating form. This type of brain injury usually involves severe structural disruption of the axons throughout all portions of the brain. While these severe types of head injury are seen most commonly in vehicle accidents, they have also been reported in Alpine skiers. Victims of severe diffuse axonal injury become unconscious immediately upon impact at the time of the traumatic event, and the unconsciousness may persist for many weeks. These patients also have persistent and often permanent brain stem signs as severe as decorticate (flaccid) or decerebrate (rigid) posturing as well as cortical neurologic dysfunctions.

Focal brain injuries are frequently encountered in sports, including Alpine skiing. As mentioned above, the focal brain injuries include various hematomas as well as cerebral contusions. These various focal brain injuries often occur in concert.

Subdural hematomas usually occur following the rupture of the bridging veins that traverse from the brain to the dural venous sinuses. The venous rupture occurs after an impact injury to the head. The clinical signs exhibited by the victim are determined by the severity of the head injury and the speed at which the hematoma expands. These patients usually are afflicted with hemiparesis (muscle weakness affecting one side of the body) as well as a disparity in the size of the pupils of the eyes.

If the meningeal arteries are ruptured as a direct result of a blow to the skull, epidural hematomas are likely to ensue. Skull fractures are the most common pathogenic mechanism of epidural hematoma formation. Classically with epidural hematomas, there is an immediate loss of consciousness following the traumatic impact which has produced the skull fracture. The victim may be fully lucid during a transient period of recovery, but as the hematoma enlarges, neurologic symptoms to include headache and lethargy develop. It should be noted that some patients with epidural hematoma do not lose consciousness for several minutes to hours after the injury, while others remain unconscious from the time of the injury.

Intracerebral hematomas are homogeneous collections of blood within the brain. This type of hematoma can result from various causes including penetrating wounds.

Finally, cerebral contusions are represented by bruising of the brain tissue. If these injuries occur at the site of impact, they are referred to as coup lesions, but if the bruising occurs at the side opposite to the point of impact, the lesions are referred to as contrecoup. The contrecoup lesion usually occurs at the time of impact at the end of an acceleration–deceleration injury. Such an injury would occur in an Alpine skier whose head collided with a stationary object resulting in an abrupt deceleration.

Risk factors

Based on various reports, it appears that the overall injury rate for Alpine skiing has remained fairly constant. However, the frequency of certain types of injuries has changed. For example, for every 100 patients who have skiing injuries which require orthopedic treatment, there are five to 10 skiers who sustain injuries to the neurological system. More recently, Harris has noted a steady increase in multiple severe injuries, especially those which involve head and spinal trauma as well as internal chest and abdominal injuries. He concludes that Alpine ski injuries are becoming similar in nature to high-velocity injuries seen in vehicular accidents.

In the series reported by Harris, of the 347 Alpine skiers who sustained a concussion, 34 (about 10%) required major cranial surgery. The skier mortality rate in this study approached 2%. No sudden death of an unexplained nature was observed in that series, and all deaths were directly attributable to the traumatic episode. In a report by Morrow, 16 deaths in Alpine skiers were reported to have occurred over seven ski seasons in Vermont. Based on their information, they calculated that there was one death per 1.5 million Alpine skiing days. Nearly all of these cases resulted in the death of the victim within the first 24 h. In another report by some of the same authors, there is a description of a syndrome referred to as "malignant cerebral edema." In that syndrome, it is believed that the compliance of the brain tissue has been previously compromised by a traumatic episode, and during a secondary episode of craniocerebral trauma there is sudden cerebral swelling. This swelling is probably due to a rapid increase in intracerebral blood. The result is usually either death or development of a chronic vegetative state under rather vague circumstances.

Harris describes the two basic types of ski accidents which occur during Alpine skiing as falls and collisions. In general, falls tend to result in injuries to the extremities. Collisions, on the other hand, may injure almost any part of the body. Collisions clearly are the most common source of head and spinal injuries in Alpine skiers. The most serious collisions were those that involved the skier hitting trees, boulders, ski lift equipment, and other skiers.

Virtually all authors agree that the two primary contributing factors to Alpine skiing accidents which produce head injuries are excessive speed and skiing out of control. Interestingly, two major improvements within the recreational ski industry have probably actually increased the risk and likelihood of serious head injuries in Alpine skiers. These marked improvements include ski slope grooming techniques and marked technical advances in the design and manufacture of skis, bindings, and ski boots. In each case, these marked improvements have permitted skiers to go down the slope at much higher speeds (probably by as much as 15–20%) and consequently this speed markedly enhances the likelihood of the loss of control. In fact, Morrow reported that of the 16 deaths in their study, 15 of the fatal injuries were actually witnessed, and in all of these cases the skiers were described as being out of control when the traumatic episode occurred.

In the report by Morrow, it did not appear that the ski equipment contributed significantly to any of the accidents. Most reports which do discuss the involvement of equipment in Alpine ski accidents involving head injuries are quick to point out that rarely, if ever, are helmets or other protective head gear worn by recreational skiers. This one item alone is estimated to prevent a large percentage of serious or lethal head injuries in Alpine skiers.

Fatigue also seems to be a risk factor in ski accidents. Harris and Morrow report that the majority of the serious head injuries occur late in the day following a full day of skiing. Likewise, in competitive skiers most of the serious injuries occur in the latter part of the race. Morrow also found that a number of the fatal head injuries occurred in skiers who were reported to have been tired from a long drive to the ski slope the night before or who reportedly had been up late the prior evening.

Age also seems to be a risk factor in serious head injuries in Alpine skiers. Virtually all of the published reports indicate that the majority of the serious head injuries occur in skiers between the ages of 16 and 25 years. The various reports indicate that this age group comprises about 50–70% of all of the seriously head-injured skiers. Furthermore, Harris reported that male skier deaths in this age group outnumbered female skier deaths by a ratio of 5 : 1. Drugs and alcohol did not appear to be a significant factor in any of the reports on head injuries in Alpine skiers. Harris reported that aerial maneuvers were a common source of serious neurologic injuries in skiers in his study, especially the 16–25-year-old males. In most of the cases reported, there was an inadequate or uncontrolled landing with the neck and back in a vulnerable position of abrupt flexion. The most common serious injuries which he reported were compound depressed skull fractures with intracranial hematomas. There were also a number of spinal cord injuries at the cervicothoracic or the thoracolumbar junction.

Other factors frequently mentioned include poor or inadequate training for the type of skiing performed. Coincident with the inadequate training is the use of inappropriate equipment for the ski activity. Poorly designed or prepared downhill ski courses have also been implicated in some serious head injuries in Alpine skiers. As previously mentioned, an almost universal absence of appropriate protective head gear is a major factor which contributes to the serious head injuries. And finally, many recreational ski areas have inadequate or suboptimal first aid, triage, or evacuation and transportation mechanisms.

Injury recognition and immediate care

When an Alpine skier with a potential or a known head injury is encountered, cautious actions must be taken to assure that no further injuries to the brain or spinal cord are produced. Prior to moving the injured skier, the "ABCs" of primary assessment should be conducted. That is, the observer should determine that the victim has a patent airway, that the patient is breathing spontaneously, and that the patient has a heartbeat. If the observer determines that there is pulmonary or cardiac arrest, cardiopulmonary resuscitation (CPR) should be begun after carefully moving the patient into the proper position for its administration. During any movement or positioning of the victim, the head and neck must be carefully stabilized. At that point the CPR provider should reestablish that the victim has a patent airway before beginning CPR using established methods. Maintenance of the respiratory and cardiac functions helps to assure that cerebral oxygenation will be maintained and that further ischemic injury to the brain will be minimized or prevented.

The level of consciousness of the head-injured

skier is the best and most important indicator of the severity of the brain trauma. Any neurologic evaluations at the site of injury should be brief, but they should at least assess and determine the level of consciousness. One of the most rapid and meaningful evaluations of mental status is the one proposed by the American College of Surgeons. That examination is referred to routinely by its moniker AVPU. The AVPU technique is based on the following four questions. Is the patient alert (A)? If not alert, does the patient respond to verbal (V) stimuli? If not responsive to verbal commands, is the patient responsive to painful (P) or noxious stimuli such as pinching a toe or finger? Or is the patient unresponsive (U) to all stimuli? Other clinical indicators that can be very quickly determined at the initial examination include the size, equality, and responsiveness to light of the pupils. One should also look for clear cerebrospinal fluid leaking from the ear canal or the nose of the victim. Whether or not fluid leakage is noted, the head should be kept elevated.

A number of grading systems to help quantify the severity of brain injuries have been developed over the past several years. While all of these grading systems provide certain specific information about the head-injured patient, all of them rely on the level of consciousness as their primary indicator.

Treatment rendered to the spine- or head-injured skier on the mountain usually should be only that required to assure that no further injuries to the central nervous system are produced. Beyond assuring adequate cardiopulmonary function and careful stabilization of the back and neck, the main efforts should be aimed at evacuating the skier quickly and safely off the mountain and reaching a medical treatment facility. While not all skiers who sustain a lesser head injury require definitive treatment, the more serious injuries must receive appropriate medical attention. Any skier who is head-injured and remains unconscious for more than a few minutes should be evacuated to a hospital for a full neurological examination and observation. If the skier appears to have a focal brain injury with hemiparesis, hemisensory loss, or hyperreflexia, the observer should consider this situation an emergency. These clinical signs would lead one to suspect intracerebral hematoma or cerebral contusion as described above. No delays in evacuation of these victims can be tolerated without the likelihood of the brain injury becoming permanent or lethal.

Some head-injured skiers may not be rendered unconscious, but they may have various post-traumatic neurologic symptoms to include headache, dizziness, blurred vision, or impaired memory. These patients also should be transported to a medical treatment facility where a complete neurologic examination can be completed and necessary observation accomplished. Head-injured skiers who experience any form of seizure should also be afforded the same treatment and observation.

Any skier suspected of having a skull fracture of any magnitude should also be provided with a detailed neurological examination. A primary indication of skull fracture is the presence of an observable or a palpable malalignment of the bony calvarium. Other indicators of skull fracture, as described above, include cerebrospinal fluid leakage from the ear canals or the nose, hematomas behind the ears, and marked hemorrhagic or ecchymotic areas in the periorbital region.

The definitive treatment of these serious to severe brain injuries frequently requires extensive and highly sophisticated neurological surgery. A description of these surgical techniques is beyond the scope of this chapter.

Prevention of injuries

Essentially all ski injuries, and especially those involving the head, can be related to either the skier, the ski equipment, or the skiing environment. Therefore, virtually all skiing accidents are preventable.

Various authors have provided recommendations of methods to prevent head injuries in Alpine skiers, but both Harris and Lehman have taken a practical approach to this problem. Both authors emphasize the need for improved safety education as a part of the ski school program. The early emphasis on safety education and training would alert the new skiers from their very beginning to the potential risks of injury in this sport. This early emphasis on safety might favorably influence the incidence of serious preventable ski injuries, especially to the head. Part of the safety education should discourage amateur participation in high-risk activities such as competitive racing and aerial maneuvers (Fig. 8.1).

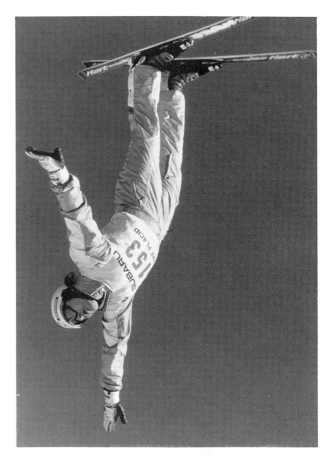

Fig. 8.1 A world-class free-style skier performing an aerial maneuver. Notice how the head, neck, and back are exposed to possible severe injury if an untoward landing should occur. © Sports File Sports Photography/D. Jenne.

Proper physical conditioning, especially in the occasional skier, might have important ramifications as well. Enhanced musculoskeletal conditioning might help to minimize some of the risk factors associated with fatigue as well as skiing out of control.

Slope design and landscaping should consider neurologic safety. Ski slopes, and especially those used for competitive Alpine events, should be designed with sufficiently clear areas around them so that the skiers have less chance of hitting stationary objects. The use of nylon nets, hay bales, and foam-filled bags adjacent to fixed solid objects has become increasingly more common (Fig. 8.2).

Because many of the head injuries in Alpine skiers

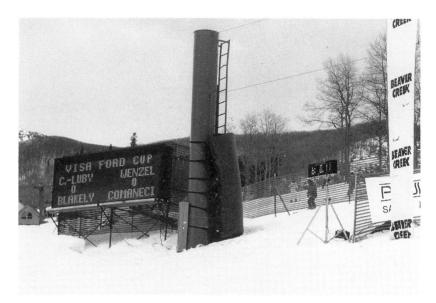

Fig. 8.2 A competitive Alpine ski course designed with maximum consideration for safety. Nylon nets and foam-filled bays protect the skiers from direct contact with stationary objects.

require immediate medical attention, it is essential that the ski area operators develop efficient and effective mechanisms for the rapid evaluation and evacuation of neurologically injured skiers. Part of this overall organization must include the cooperation of a medical treatment facility with advanced capabilities in neurologic diagnostic and treatment techniques. Depending on the location of the ski area, part of this mechanism should include a provision for air evacuation to the medical facility. Additionally, ski patrol personnel should be trained and educated to recognize many of the injuries described above so that they can hasten the evacuation of the patient. As Harris states, these on-mountain personnel must be trained to "look beyond the leg."

Virtually all discussions of injury prevention include improved equipment, and special emphasis is usually placed on the wearing of helmets (Fig. 8.3). While most of these recommendations for the use of helmets are rather anecdotal, Ommaya has addressed this problem in a scientific and technical manner. He points out that helmets protect the head by two mechanisms: energy absorption and load distribution. The amount of energy absorbed is based on the thickness of the helmet and the component materials. With the helmets currently available, the scalp and skull are protected against an impact that would equate to a speed of about 32 km/h (20 mile/h). Likewise,

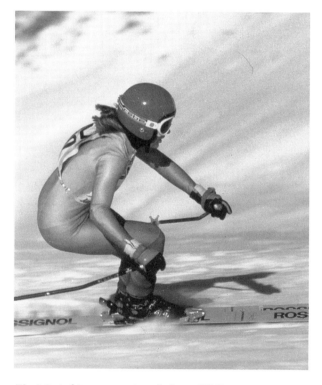

Fig. 8.3 A ski racer wearing a helmet. While most competitive skiers now routinely wear helmets, it is rare to see this precaution practiced by recreational skiers. Many experts believe that wearing helmets might significantly decrease the number of serious head injuries among Alpine skiers.

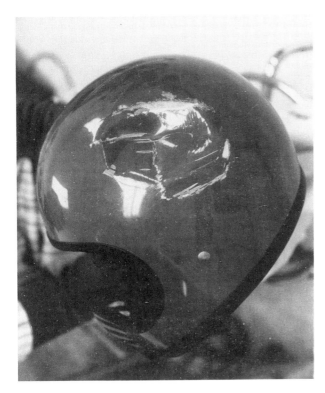

Fig. 8.4 A damaged ski helmet. The ski racer wearing this helmet lost control, skied off the course, fell, and landed head first against a rock. In spite of the extensive damage to the helmet, the skier sustained no head injury.

the brain is protected against focal contusions. On the other hand, load distribution protection of the head is based upon conversion of penetrating focal loads to more broadly distributed loads (Fig. 8.4). The maximum limitations of this mechanism are similar to those described for energy absorption. Consequently, the more diffuse injuries to the brain may be only minimally mitigated by helmets, especially when the velocity at the time of injury exceeds 32 km/h (20 mile/h). However while helmets prevent injuries, they do not prevent accidents.

Rehabilitation and return to sport

Physical rehabilitation following severe neurologic injuries is an art and science of its own. No attempt to describe those specific rehabilitative techniques will be provided in this chapter. One might say, however, that safety education should be a part of any rehabili-

tative program for head-injured skiers prior to their return to sport.

The criteria and timing for resumption of participation in Alpine skiing remains somewhat debatable. As Harris has pointed out, the neurologic risks of advanced Alpine skiing make it essentially equivalent in risk to contact sports such as football. The timing for the return to downhill skiing relates most closely to the severity of the original injury, the mechanism of injury, and the extent of involvement of associated central nervous system injuries.

The most significant debate on when to return to skiing seems to involve those patients in which the head injury was mild or moderate. If the victim exhibits amnesia, then resumption of skiing should be delayed until all neurologic functions are normal. Harris has suggested that the best way to determine the occurrence of amnesia and its duration is to ask both of these two key questions:
1 What is the last thing you remember before getting hurt?
2 What is the next thing you remember?
These two questions are likely to provide a significant amount of information regarding the amnesia.

When there is an obvious, severe head injury, the victim should be forced to terminate the sporting activity and to remain under observation until all neurologic dysfunction has resolved. Coaches and medical care personnel must cooperate and enforce the cessation of activities.

Norrell has developed a set of guidelines for when an athlete should return to participation in a contact sport or high-risk sport following a neurologic injury. While these guidelines were not developed specifically for Alpine skiing, the same conditions apply since the competitive or advanced skier is at high risk of repeated neurologic trauma. With specific emphasis on head injuries, Norrell has stated that an athlete should not resume the sport on the same day if the athlete sustained a concussion with any residual effects such as retrograde amnesia, confusion, headache, or unexplained behavior. The skier should consider not returning to skiing for the remainder of the season if there has been any seizure activity following the head trauma. This guideline holds true whether the seizure activity is single, multiple, focal, or generalized. Norrell also emphasizes that special attention should be given to determining the etiology of the seizure activity to exclude any pre-existing brain abnormalities. He also suggests that the skier not return for the remainder of the season after a post-concussion syndrome in which there has been persistent headache, dizziness, vertigo, irritability, inability to concentrate, impaired memory, and fatigue. Further, he strongly suggests that skiers not return to their sport at all if there have been repeated concussions with recurrent postconcussion syndrome. Any intracranial surgery as a result of the head trauma is also an indication not to return to skiing. And finally, Norrell recommends that all contact sports be forbidden if the victim continues to experience symptomatic neurologic abnormalities of almost any kind that do not resolve over a period of approximately 1 year.

Nonetheless, Norrell emphasizes that careful reassessment be the primary basis upon which individual decisions are made regarding the return to participation after neurologic injury. Furthermore, hard and fast rules are both difficult to make and difficult to enforce.

Conclusion

Head injuries in Alpine skiers are a significant source of morbidity and mortality. Emphasis must be placed on prevention of these injuries by insisting on safety training at a very early stage of the skier's career. Proper activity and use of equipment in Alpine skiing can also help to prevent injuries. Head-injured skiers must receive prompt professional attention following their injury to help minimize further brain deterioration. Professional consultation must be a portion of any decision for the skier to return to skiing following a severe head injury or post-concussion syndrome.

Recommended reading

Gennarelli, T.A. (1987) Cerebral concussion and diffuse brain injuries. In Cooper, P.R. (ed.) *Head Injury*. Baltimore: Williams & Wilkins, pp. 108–124.

Harris, J.B. (1983) Neurological injuries in winter sports. *Phys. Sportsmed.* **11**:111–122.

Harris, J.B. (1989) Neurological injuries in skiing and winter sports in America. In Jordan, B.D., Tsairis, P. & Warren, R.F. (eds) *Sports Neurology*. Rockville: Aspen Publishers, pp. 295–304.

Lehman, L.B. (1986) Neurologic injuries from winter sporting accidents: how they happen and how to minimize them. *Postgrad. Med.* **80**:92–98.

Norrell, H. (1971) The neurosurgeon's responsibility in the prevention of sports injuries. *Clin. Neurosurg.* **19**:212–214.

Chapter 9
Eyes

Both recreational and ski racing may present problems for the eyes. The eyes must be protected, particularly when ski racing, because when a fall occurs there is always the potential of striking the eye and producing either deep damage to the globe or scratching the cornea. The eyes also need protection from both snow and wind. If the skier has an accident which involves the eyes and then has the sensation that there is a corneal scratch or any residual eye pain, the eye should be patched to protect it, and the skier should be taken directly to an ophthalmologist. Scratches on the cornea are painful and will disturb vision for a while, but most recover well provided they are attended to. A more severe eye injury requires immediate treatment by a qualified person, thus transport to a facility and specialist must be done immediately. Corneal freezing may occasionally occur in skiers but is seen much more often in the cross-country participant as opposed to the Alpine skier. Protective goggles should avoid this situation, but if there is any suspicion of corneal damage, protect the eye and see an ophthalmologist immediately.

Protection of the eyes is best achieved by using either goggles or appropriate sunglasses. The goggles must fit well and be made of a substance that will not shatter on impact. Shatter-proof glass is used in most glasses and can be used for skiing even though its optical clarity is somewhat reduced compared to the norm. Polycarbonate is a light impact-resistant polymer, now used in many glasses and goggles and will be used more in the future, particularly as its optical clarity is gradually improved.

Another problem for a skier's eye relates to the sun's rays. On many days the eyes will need protection from the sun's ultraviolet rays. Virtually all skiers would be more comfortable using sunglasses or goggles to decrease the sun's glare which is accentuated by the white snowy background. While sunglasses make the eyes more comfortable, they do also serve another function. There is the possibility, particularly at higher altitudes, of sustaining damage to the retina of the eye from long exposure to the bright sun rays. Sunglasses should be used which block virtually all of the ultraviolet B rays and approximately 60% of the ultraviolet A rays. This should give good protection for the eyes.

Being unprotected on the slopes during bright sunshine for a long period of time can actually produce solar blindness due to the ultraviolet solar radiation. This may cause pitting of the cornea and disruption of the epithelial surface. Rarely retinal damage will occur. Symptoms develop within hours of exposure and there is generalized swelling and erythema of the eyelid and/or cornea. This is a major ophthalmologic emergency and treatment will include drops to dilate the pupil, coverage of the affected eye, and in many instances antibiotics.

Sunglasses reduce the intensity of light in various ways. Mirrored glasses can reduce the intensity by reflecting part of the light so that it does not actually enter the eyes. Polarized glasses will greatly reduce glare, usually without reducing the normal light to any significant extent. Tinted glasses filter out certain of the colors of the spectrum and by this reduce light absorption. There are also photosensitive or photo chromatic glasses which have lenses that darken when the light is bright outside and lighten when it is cloudy.

One must be aware that on overcast days, goggles may cut out some sunlight thus diminishing the ability of the skier to follow the terrain carefully. On such days the lack of sunshine makes it difficult to pick up bumps and gullies because of the lack of contrast. Tinted lenses may help. This may be a particular problem for the racer who is trying to see ski tracks and the upcoming gates as quickly as possible. However, racers will need goggles or glasses because conditions including sun, wind, or snow may make it difficult to see while going fast.

Goggles may present a problem because of fogging of the lens system. Most try to solve this by some type of ventilation which does not always work despite most manufacturer's claims. In ski racing, visibility is critical and the racer must be sure that goggles are working properly. If the goggles are dependent upon ventilation by using holes around the periphery, these must be clear of snow, debris, and so on. Other goggles are built with a double lens and a sealed thermal barrier in between which is supposed to prevent fogging. Certain others have anti-fogging coats on the inner lens. The authors advise the ski racer to be aware of the possible methods to avoid fogging, but it is best to rely on your own practical experience or that of friends as to which particular set of goggles and system will work best for racing. For the ski racer well fitted, well-functioning goggles with the appropriate lenses are a necessity.

Chapter 10

Neck

Neck injuries are uncommon in skiing, but those that occur may have potentially serious or even fatal consequences. These injuries occur either as the result of a fall or collision, and the more serious ones will be the consequence of high-speed injuries. Major damage to the neck usually results from a flexion injury with force applied to the head and transmitted to the vertebral column.

Recognizing a neck injury may be difficult because of two circumstances.

1 The patient may have received a concomitant head injury, be unconscious, and unable to tell the examiner of the nature or extent of his or her injuries.

2 Although the patient may have neck pain, he or she may not be aware of the severity of the injury, particularly if there is no immediate resultant paralysis or weakness of any extremity.

With the unconscious patient one must always assume the possibility of a head or spinal injury and treat the skier as if that were a probability. This means that enough competent help must be available to move the skier on to a firm stretcher or transport board. The head and neck must be handled by the person with the most experience in dealing with such injuries, and the head and neck should be kept in as near normal an anatomical position as possible. It is best to have the head initially held by hand and then perhaps cradled in some fashion with a pillow or available soft goods. If the head is turned to one side in an abnormal posture, it would be best, particularly with the unconscious skier, to put the patient on the transport board with the head cradled in that position. If there is an available neck brace or collar that may be very carefully applied.

If this accident occurs on a mountain during a big race, there should be aid standing by, ready to evacu-ate the racer from the scene of injury. In other instances at the lower levels of racing or recreational skiing, the patient may have to wait to be transported down the mountain, and this puts the ski patrol and toboggan operators on their mettle. With the unconscious patient the possible extent of injuries are unknown, and any damage beyond what has already happened must be minimized.

With patients having head or neck trauma, respiratory distress may occur and an open airway must be maintained. Cold and resultant hypothermia may be a problem for these skiers, because it often takes a considerable period of time to transport the patient off the mountain. The patient must be kept warm.

A basic concept for anybody having a suspected neck injury is "assume the worst but do your best." Once the patient has been moved off the mountain, he or she should be taken to the closest available properly equipped facility for someone with a spinal injury. If this is a ski area with a doctor at the base of the slope, transportation should be waiting, ready to go as soon as the patient and toboggan arrive. The area doctor should do a quick examination to determine vital signs and may decide to accompany the patient to the local hospital. Somebody should travel with the patient to be sure that the head and neck are properly positioned.

Once the patient arrives at the hospital, a full physical examination is carefully performed. Anteroposterior and lateral X-rays, including all of the cervical spine, will be performed, and the treatment following that is dependent upon the extent of injuries. With a cervical fracture, dislocation, facet subluxation, or any extremity weakness or paralysis, the initial care is likely to involve putting some external fixation tongs in the skull to control the head and neck. It is, however, beyond the scope of this chapter to give definitive treatment of major neck injuries. Even radiographs may be difficult to interpret and a unilateral facet subluxation can easily be missed by the uninitiated. With a neck injury it becomes mandatory that the patient see an orthopedic surgeon or neurosurgeon with experience in cervical trauma.

Some patients will have lesser trauma and will simply appear to have a painful stiff neck. These patients will have no weakness, paralysis, or major symptoms. They can be treated with either a soft collar or a Philadelphia splint while appropriate X-rays

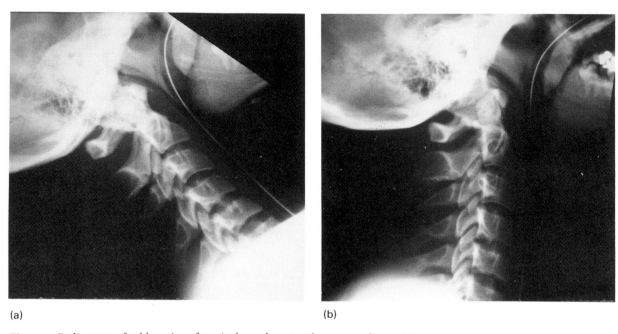

(a)   (b)

Fig. 10.1 Radiograms of subluxation of cervical vertebrae 3 and 4, seen on flexion (a) but not on extension (b).

are taken. It is much better to overtreat an initial neck injury than to undertreat.

Fractures of the vertebra, even a compression fracture or fracture of the anterior lip, may occur without paralysis. With treatment these may eventually heal, producing a stable neck which is consistent with later skiing. However, any neck injury, fracture, fracture dislocation, or subluxation, must be evaluated for stability. Generally, flexion and extension films and in some instances cine studies in flexion and extension may have to be done to determine the stability of a neck following the acute phase of the injury (Fig. 10.1). Anybody suffering a major injury to the neck such as described above or who has a spinal stabilization procedure must receive advice from the specialist as to whether or not they should continue further skiing or ski racing. Once a spinal stabilization procedure has been done, there is some loss of the normal energy-absorbing capacity of the spine, and this raises doubts as to whether one should be involved in ski racing again. It is best to judge this on an individual basis.

Neck sprains

Other less serious injuries do occur, and the majority turn out to be a sprain of the neck muscles. This is usually the result of a fall with twisting of the head, and while the skier recognizes that there is pain, there is no loss of function. Often, the racer simply continues racing or practicing but hours later, or the next morning, may find there is a great deal more neck pain. With pain, muscle spasm often occurs and motion of the neck becomes decreased. Routine X-rays including an anteroposterior, lateral, and obliques of the cervical spine are then indicated. If these are negative, the diagnosis is likely to be a cervical sprain.

Acutely, ice applied to the neck is helpful in reducing spasm, although sometimes it is an unpleasant sensation for the skier. A soft collar may be worn for several days to decrease pain. It is important however, not to use the collar for a long period of time but rather to start rehabilitation of the neck muscles. We usually start with gentle range of motion neck exercises going to the right, to the left, and forward flexion, staying within the limits of pain. Extension is more likely to cause pain, and so this should not be included in the initial phase. Exercises should be performed on an hourly or every 2-h basis, completing five to 10 repetitions staying within the limits of pain and trying to achieve a little bit more motion each day.

Once motion is regained, then the skier should start strengthening exercises of the neck muscles. It is not easy to do, but resistance can be provided by the skier's own hand or by a bungee cord which encircles the head and is held by the other hand as the neck turns. Chronic neck pain is often the result of inadequate rehabilitation, both in terms of gaining range of motion and strength. It is a mistake to depend upon the use of a collar for an extended period of time as this leads to muscle atrophy and eventually increased problems.

A nonsteroidal anti-inflammatory drug may be helpful during the first few days to relieve pain and spasm. By relieving pain initially, skiers may feel that they are better than they really are physiologically, and the skier may be tempted to go back too soon.

Most neck sprains resolve in a 7–14-day period, although rehabilitation of the muscles may take longer to resume normal strength.

Neck injuries occur primarily as the result of falls and collisions particularly at high speeds. While the ski racer's helmet is helpful in decreasing the impact forces to the skull, it does not do much for the neck. Some skiers who survive a head injury with a helmet may end up with a neck injury, not because of the helmet but because of the force involved. Neck injuries are less likely in routine recreational skiing but are seen in inverted aerial free-style competitions. There really is no protective device which gives adequate help for these people who are at risk whilst performing inverted aerials. Lift area operators have tried to protect against collisions versus fixed objects such as lift towers on ski runs, but there is no protection for the out of control skier who goes off the trail into a tree. Lack of control and speed are the major factors in neck injuries.

Chapter 11

Spine, thorax, abdomen, and pelvis

Injuries to the spine, thorax, abdomen, and pelvis are relatively uncommon in skiing and ski racing. They are far less frequent than injuries to the extremities but when they occur they can be very serious. The reason for this is that injuries to these four areas occur as the result of impact, such as a fall or collision against the ground, tree, lift tower, and so on. The faster the ski racer is going at the time of impact, the more severe the injury will be. These injuries are not related to equipment but to skiing skills and control.

Spine

Injuries to the thoracic and lumbar spine have the same potential for disaster that a neck injury has. There are two possible ways for a racer to injure the thoracic or lumbar spine. The first is by going out of control and hitting a stationary object such as a tree, lift tower, and so on. Such a collision could cause a fracture or dislocation of the spine and the resultant injury would depend upon the object hit, the speed the racer was traveling, and the area of the back which was impacted. The second way that an injury could happen would be for the skier to go off a bump or hit a compression the wrong way and land heavily and awkwardly on the ground. This type of injury is much more likely to cause a compression fracture of the vertebrae.

In either instance the severity of the injury is usually obvious as the skier complains of back pain and in rare instances paralysis or weakness below the level of injury. The short- and long-term goals are the same: trying to avoid any injury to the spinal cord and to minimize any damage that has already occurred due to the accident. The skier must be handled with maximal care for the spine as he or she is put on the toboggan or basket which will take the patient off the race

course. The whole body must be moved as a unit. No flexion, extension, lateral bending, or rotation of the body is allowed. All care should be taken in getting the skier stabilized for removal off the hill. Then the skier should be taken immediately to an area medical facility to obtain X-rays of the entire spine if possible.

Once the diagnosis has been made of a fracture or fracture dislocation of the spine, a treatment plan can then be formulated. This plan would depend upon a number of factors, including whether or not the fracture is stable or unstable, how much of a vertebrae is compressed, and the presence or absence of paralysis.

Fractures or fracture dislocations which are judged unstable will be best handled by surgery and stabilization by one of the many instrumentation techniques available. A stable fracture can be handled with a period of bed rest and then some type of brace or back support. It is even possible that if the compression of the vertebrae is minimal that no support would be needed while the fracture is healing.

The question of being able to ski race again depends on many factors, including whether or not there is any paralysis and whether or not the spinal column had to be stabilized and fused. In those instances where there is only a slight compression fracture of the vertebrae, there is no reason to believe that the racer could not return once everything has healed. When the injury is more severe and needs operative stabilization, any decision about return would have to be made on an individual basis, but this might very well herald the end of ski racing for that particular individual.

Thorax

Injuries to the thorax may range from a contusion of the ribs to fractures of the ribs with damage to the underlying lungs. Injuries to the thorax are not uncommon in ski racing as a result of hitting the ground or less commonly, as a result of hitting a stationary object. In most instances this represents a simple contusion of the rib cage which can be treated symptomatically. However, if there is acute pain, and particularly when there is any local tenderness in the area of the rib cage, a fracture of the ribs must be suspected. If there is any bleeding from the mouth after an injury to the rib cage, that would be a clear indication of a contusion of the underlying lungs and emergency treatment is mandatory.

When there is a suspicion of rib fracture or rib fracture plus damage to the lungs, the skier must be taken to an area hospital. X-rays should be taken which will determine the presence or absence of fracture and also determine if there is a collapse of the lungs which would necessitate the insertion of a chest tube to reinflate the lungs.

Treatment of fractured ribs or even a contusion of the ribs is relatively difficult. The major worry is the pain that results, and this is only significantly decreased with medication. Strapping of the ribs is not particularly effective and in many instances seems to be worse than the condition itself. One problem for patients with fractured ribs is that they breathe very shallowly to avoid pain, thus the lungs are not properly inflated, creating a risk for pneumonia. Fortunately, in most young healthy patients this phase is over relatively quickly and the risk of developing pneumonia is unlikely.

With a contusion, the skier can usually return to racing when the pain is gone and a good deep breath is taken without pain. With rib fractures, that usually requires the fracture's healing and the racer being able to take a good deep breath without causing pain.

Abdomen

Abdominal injuries happen the same way as injuries to the thorax, which is usually by a direct blow. These are less common and the consequences are usually not severe. However, serious injury could result when a fast travelling racer suddenly hits a tree or lift tower and thus sustains damage to one of the internal organs. The most likely internal organ to be injured is the spleen which is located in the left upper quadrant of the abdomen. Generally, anybody producing an injury severe enough to cause a rupture or bleeding into the splenic capsule will have had a severe fall

which would necessitate careful examination by a physician. Tenderness in the upper outer quadrant of the abdomen would indicate the possibility of damage to the spleen. If there was major damage, the spleen might literally be ruptured and this would cause internal bleeding and a subsequent fall in blood pressure. In some rare instances there is simply a crack in the spleen which produces bleeding in the capsule and there may be a late subsequent fall in blood pressure from internal bleeding. This is why skiers who sustain a major impact injury to the abdomen should be watched for a period of time (24–48 h) by medical personnel. Injuries of this kind are relatively rare but if they happen, they are the result of high-speed injuries and collision.

Pelvic fractures

Pelvic fractures are uncommon in skiing. They are likely to occur only at very high speeds and, in most instances, are the result of hitting a fixed object. A pelvic fracture is a serious injury and may be life endangering because of the great amount of bleeding that can occur from the fracture surfaces. Any skier who has a pelvic fracture will have severe pain immediately and will be unable to stand. Cardiovascular collapse can occur quickly because of bleeding from the bones of the pelvis, which means that the patient must be quickly transported to an emergency facility which has blood available plus the other elements for treating cardiovascular collapse.

A major consideration for any skier who is suspected of having a pelvic injury is to assure careful handling and removal of the patient from the ski slope. With a pelvic fracture, all consideration must be given to careful handling of the skier onto a toboggan and from there to an emergency evacuation vehicle and to a hospital.

Chapter 12

Upper extremities

During the past 30 years, ski center statistics have revealed a gradual downward trend in the incidence of recreational skiing injuries. The current data suggest an injury incidence somewhere between two and four injuries per 1000 skier days. Of this, it appears that upper extremity injuries account for 1.06 injuries per 1000 skier days. These data concerning the upper extremity are probably under-reported since some injuries are not severe enough to cause injured skiers to seek immediate mountain-based medical treatment. This is particularly true with upper extremity ski injuries since in many instances, the skier would be able to return home because of a lesser disability than a lower extremity injury might cause.

Table 12.1 Upper extremity injuries. With permission from Carr *et al.* (1981)

Diagnosis	No.	%
Thumb UCL–MCP sprain/fracture	162	37.0
Shoulder soft tissue injury	79	18.0
Shoulder dislocation	39	8.9
Contusion of arm or hand	39	8.9
Metacarpal fracture	22	5.0
Wrist sprain	15	3.4
Thumb phalanx fracture	15	3.4
Proximal humerus fracture	13	3.0
Laceration with suture	13	3.0
Distal radius fracture	12	2.7
Clavicle fracture	11	2.5
Dislocation of sprain–IP thumb	11	2.5
Miscellaneous	7	1.6
Total	438	99.9

IP, interphalangeal; MCP, metocarpophalangeal; UCL, ulnar collateral ligament.

While lower extremity ski injuries have decreased largely secondarily to equipment modifications, upper extremity injuries have increased in relative frequency. Hand and shoulder injuries account for the vast majority of this increase. Carr listed the most frequent upper extremity injuries (Table 12.1) for recreational skiers; these are also probably applicable for racers. The vast majority of upper extremity injuries occur as the result of falls, with the rest resulting from a collision with an object or another individual.

Thumb/ulnar ligament injury

The ulnar collateral ligament (UCL) of the thumb may account for up to 20% of all reported ski injuries (Fig. 12.1). Most authorities feel that this injury is under-reported, particularly by recreational skiers because the initial disability is not as great as for other common injuries such as the knee. For the racer, the disability from the thumb UCL injury is considerable and it is likely that we would have an early reporting of such as injury from the racer. The damage to the thumb usually occurs during a fall on the outstretched hand, usually with the ski pole held in the palm. The pole forces the thumb into extension and radial deviation at the metacarpophalangeal (MCP) joint. The same injury can occur without the pole as the hand hits the ground in the outstretched position while the skier is trying to cushion the fall. The severity of the injury ranges from no instability at the MCP point (grade 1 sprain) to partial instability (grade 2 sprain) to total instability (grade 3 sprain). A grade 3 UCL disruption often requires surgical repair to ensure optimal recovery.

While the skier may have some pain in the thumb following the initial fall, pain may not be a real problem until the next day when swelling has occurred overnight, causing more dysfunction and pain. The skier usually feels stiffness and instability is an uncommon initial complaint. In many instances, even with a third-degree sprain, the skier may not seek early treatment which accounts for some of the late surgical repairs that have to be performed. However, for the racer, the inability to firmly grip the pole will probably make him or her seek aid early.

Stener described the essential lesion in grade 3 injuries, stating that the adductor pollicis aponeurosis becomes interposed between the two torn ends of

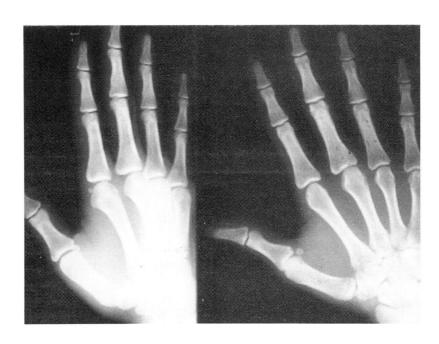

Fig. 12.1 Radiogram of an avulsion fracture of the base of the proximal thumb phalanx with ulnar collateral ligament instability.

the UCL. Thus, normal healing is prevented. This lack of healing would result in laxity at the MCP joint and with radial stress on the thumb as occurs in pinching between the index finger and thumb or even by holding a ski pole, both pain and weakness result. It requires an index of clinical suspicion to make the initial correct diagnosis. Generally, the racer has tenderness over the ulnar aspect of the MCP joint. The thumb should be gently stressed, both in extension and in partial flexion, and the amount of radial valgus compared on the injured side to the uninjured side. A difference of 20° or more makes one suspect that there is a grade 3 sprain. Routine X-rays of the thumb should always be done since approximately 20% of these injuries show an avulsed bony fragment, usually at the base of the proximal phalanx. Stress radiographs which show greater than 45° of laxity at the MCP joint always indicate a grade 3 sprain.

Treatment of UCL sprains varies according to the grade of sprain. Grade 1 sprains usually require some immobilization, usually in a cast, although a splint may suffice until symptoms abate. This may be only 2–3 weeks. Alternatively, the thumb can be carefully taped or a removable splint applied. Grade 2 sprains usually have to be casted for 3–6 weeks and then protected for an additional 2–4 weeks at which time,

flexion–extension exercises are initiated. In a ski racer, it might be possible to make a specially molded plastic gauntlet which would protect the ligament during healing, but still allow the skier to hold the pole and to race.

Because of the high incidence of Stener lesions in acute grade 3 injuries, early operative repair is usually advocated. Good to excellent results can be expected in 96% of surgically treated cases. Surgery consists of accurately identifying the torn portions of the ligament and suturing them together, or alternatively, if the ligament is avulsed with or without a piece of bone from the base of the proximal phalanx, the ligament can be replaced in its anatomical position, usually with a pull-out wire. Casting is applied for 6 weeks and rehabilitation would be another 2–4 weeks, following which the skier would be expected to have a normal grip.

There has been much discussion about the prevention of ulnar collateral injuries. Some studies have implicated poles and straps as a major cause of injury and poles with molded grips have been advised. However, strapless poles and poles with molded grips have not made a significant change in the injury rate. In ski racing, it is not reasonable to place one's hand outside the ski pole strap, which is a possible way of decreasing the potential of this injury. As long as poles are used in downhill skiing and people continue to fall in a forward position, then there is the likelihood of UCL ruptures. Early recognition and treatment can be expected to restore function in a high percentage of cases. Late reconstructions do not fare as well as acute repairs, but they still have a high success rate.

Shoulder injuries

Shoulder injuries are relatively common in both ski racing and recreational skiing. They are almost always the result of falls onto snow and much less commonly, the result of a collision with a fixed object. The best index of the severity of a shoulder injury is how much pain the skier is experiencing. The location of the pain will indicate the probable diagnosis. The most severe injury would be a shoulder dislocation or a fracture either of the clavicle or humerus. A somewhat less severe injury, but one causing pain with dysfunction and a relatively long convalescence is a shoulder separation.

Shoulder dislocation

Of the shoulder injuries, anterior shoulder dislocations (Fig. 12.2) are the highest in frequency and the second most common upper extremity ski injury. The shoulder (glenohumeral joint) is the most mobile joint in the body. Stability is provided primarily by the muscles and capsular ligaments surrounding the joint. A single major traumatic event may disrupt these soft tissues and cause a shoulder dislocation. While a direct blow might force the humeral head out of the socket, it is more common for an indirect force to be the cause of anterior shoulder dislocation. If a racer falls with an arm forward and outstretched from the body, force is applied to the hand and arm and this leverage is applied to the shoulder. It may cause a rupture of the capsular ligaments and as these soft tissue restraints are torn and the force continues, the humeral head is levered out of the joint anteriorly. This usually happens as the result of a fall, but may occur as the result of a vigorous pole plant where the arm is held posterior to the body as the body moves forward and leverage pops the shoulder out. Hooking the arm on a slalom gate as the skier goes through could cause a shoulder dislocation.

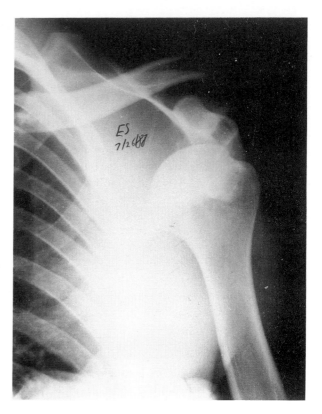

Fig. 12.2 Radiogram of anterior shoulder dislocation.

Usually a racer who has suffered a dislocation will know or have a high index of suspicion that the shoulder has gone out. They usually feel something pop and the pain is immediate and severe. This racer will resist an attempt to move the arm and will try to cradle the arm against the body. The diagnosis of an anterior shoulder dislocation often can be made on the ski slope. If a physician is on the course and immediately available, he or she may be able to apply longitudinal traction to the arm while the skier is held by someone else to provide counter-traction and the shoulder may immediately be reduced before there is significant muscle spasm. The disadvantage of doing this on the hill is that if there is any associated fracture or nerve injury which has occurred during the dislocation, this may not be initially picked up. The advantage of immediate reduction in the hands of somebody skilled is that the skier's pain is relieved quickly.

Under the usual circumstances, the skier would be taken off the hill in a toboggan with the arm carefully cradled against the body. While vascular injuries are uncommon in dislocated shoulders, the neurovascular status in the upper extremities should be noted immediately. An injury to either the axillary nerve or one of the three primary nerves going down the arm is relatively common. A quick examination should be done to check sensation and motor function of the hand and sensation over the deltoid portion of the shoulder, which is served by the axillary nerve. X-rays of the affected shoulder are taken to see if there is an associated fracture which would complicate treatment and to be sure as to whether the shoulder is located anteriorly or posteriorly.

Posterior dislocations are uncommon, so unless there is a clinical reason to suspect this, such as a lack of external rotation of the arm, an axillary view is not mandatory, although it is helpful in all shoulder injuries. With an anterior dislocation, one should try to do an immediate reduction by gentle longitudinal traction. The patient benefits from some intramuscular or intravenous sedation and the shoulder is then reduced by traction. One of the easiest and safest methods of reducing the shoulder is having the patient lie face down on a plinth with the affected arm hanging over the side. By attaching a 5–7 kg (10–15 lb) weight to the elbow, this will overcome muscle spasm and after 15 min, the weight will usually cause the shoulder to reduce itself. In some instances, gentle manipulation by the physician can be added. Following reduction, repeat X-rays and a repeat neurovascular examination are performed to verify that the anatomy has been restored and that everything is fine. The arm is then placed in a sling or sling and swathe to keep the arm by the body and to allow for soft tissue healing.

The most frequent complication of an acute traumatic anterior shoulder dislocation is recurrent instability. The age of the skier at the time of initial injury, the presence or absence of associated fractures, and perhaps, the duration of immobilization are all factors which have been correlated with recurrent dislocations. Above the age of 40, the risk of redislocation is minimal. The majority of people practising ski racing are in their teens and early twenties and the rate of recurrent dislocation is high in these groups.

One cannot categorically state how long an anterior acute shoulder dislocation should be immobilized to aid in preventing recurrent dislocations. There is tearing of the capsular soft tissues of the shoulder, and it seems reasonable to hold the shoulder for a period of 3 weeks to allow that soft tissue to heal. The shoulder should be held at 0° of abduction in some internal rotation. Following that, the patient has to go through a period of gentle mobilization and rehabilitation of the muscle groups around the shoulder. For a skier who has had a primary acute shoulder dislocation, the restoration of normal motion and normal strength is mandatory before allowing the skier back to ski racing. It is most important to strengthen the internal rotators since these are the muscles which bring the arm back into the body and are most protective in terms of preventing a recurrent dislocation.

Recurrent shoulder dislocations

Particularly in the young ski racer, recurrent anterior dislocations are a likely prospect. If a shoulder dislocation recurs, treat the patient symptomatically, i.e. for pain and once that pain has disappeared and mobility and strength have been restored, allow the racer to return to activity. In some instances, this treatment period would be only a few days in the sling, plus a period of time for mobilization. In other instances, it might be no more than a few days of decreased activity. Generally, the more times that the shoulder has redislocated and the less trauma it has taken to go out, the shorter the period of incapacitation will be. It is recommended that a ski racer who is suffering from recurrent shoulder dislocations have a surgical repair since the success rate is over 95%, and this could be accomplished in the off season, followed by rehabilitation and readiness for the next season.

Rotator cuff tears

One other disabling soft tissue problem of the shoulder is a tear of the rotator cuff. Fortunately, cuff tears from skiing are rare, but could occur as the result of a fall on the outstretched arm or directly on the shoulder. In the recreational skier, rotator cuff injuries are more common than in the competitive race skiers because racers are usually younger. The rotator cuff tissue in a racer is of better quality, and the incidence of cuff tears is low. The incidence of a contusion of the cuff is, however, high and it may take a few days for the physician to determine that the cuff is painful but intact, as opposed to there being a small tear of the rotator cuff.

Cuff tears cause some pain, but it is not severe. This makes diagnosis difficult because the patient, rather than complaining of pain, may have only functional loss. On the hill, the skier may be able to continue down, despite some pain in the shoulder, but if there is any question, it would be best to bandage the arm against the body and bring the skier down. With the acute injury, X-rays are taken to rule out a fracture, particularly of the greater tuberosity of the humerus. If the patient has difficulty in initiating abduction or has weakness of external rotation, a rotator cuff injury must be suspect. Most of these injuries in racers will be just a contusion of the cuff, but even a small tear should be diagnosed because they respond well to early surgical management. If there is rapid improvement of abduction and strength, then a contusion is likely, but if abduction continues to be difficult and external rotation is poor, a shoulder arthrogram or arthroscopy of the shoulder is recommended. Since acute repairs of the rotator cuff do well, there is no reason not to proceed toward performing an early operation on an acute rupture of the rotator cuff. Any unexplained weakness of the arm in external rotation or abduction which follows a fall must be explained and a definitive diagnosis made.

Rehabilitation of rotator cuff injury, be it a simple contusion or a tear followed by surgery, will involve range of motion exercises plus strengthening the internal and external rotators of the shoulder plus the abductors and forward flexors.

Acromioclavicular separations

In skiing, acromioclavicular separations are less common than shoulder dislocations and happen either as the result of a fall on the outstretched arm or as the result of a direct fall on the point of the shoulder. Depending upon the force applied, a first-, second-, or third-degree (Fig. 12.3) separation of the shoulder would occur. In a first-degree separation, the coracoclavicular ligaments are intact, but there is damage to the acromioclavicular ligaments and the capsule of the acromioclavicular joint. The distal end of the clavicle is not elevated above the acromion. With a second-degree injury, the coracoclavicular ligaments

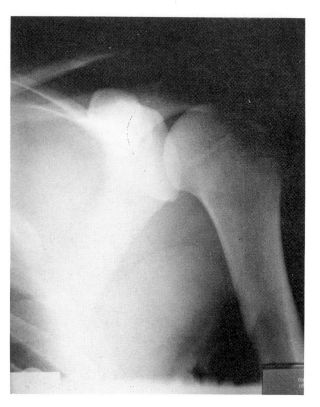

Fig. 12.3 Radiogram of a third-degree acromioclavicular separation.

are also partially torn, allowing the distal end of the clavicle to raise a bit above the acromion, and the joint surface is partially incongruous. In the third-degree separation, there is a total disruption of the coracoclavicular ligaments and the distal clavicle is elevated completely above the acromion.

With any separation of the acromioclavicular joint, the initial complaint is of pain in the acromioclavicular joint area. It hurts to move the shoulder and the racer will protect the arm. It may be possible for a racer to ski down the slope not using the affected arm by cradling that arm against the body. Most skiers would prefer to be taken down either on a lift or a toboggan, again protecting the arm against the body so further damage is not done to the acromioclavicular joint. On physical examination, there will be tenderness over the joint. If there is tenderness, but the clavicle and the acromion is at the same level, it is likely that it is only a first-degree separation; slightly elevated, it would appear to be a second-degree injury; and if the clavicle is well above the acromion, it is probably a third-degree injury. X-rays should be taken. It is advisable to use weights tied to both fore-arms as the patient stands and the X-rays are taken of both shoulders with the weights pulling the arms down. Check both the distance between the distal end of the clavicle and the acromion and the distance between the coracoid process and the acromion. By so doing, the degree of injury can be determined.

Nonoperative treatment of type 1 and type 2 acromioclavicular injuries should produce good results. The arm is immobilized in the sling for as long as there is significant tenderness. When that tenderness disappears, range of motion exercises are instituted and the skier is started back on strengthening exercises for all the shoulder girdle muscles, but particularly the trapezius. As soon as there is full range of motion and local tenderness is gone, there is no reason why the skier cannot return to full activity, including racing. A slight elevation of the clavicle above the acromion is no functional loss.

With a third-degree separation, there is a marked difference of medical opinion as to the best treatment plan. Many doctors feel that such a separation could be treated nonoperatively. Others state that the acromioclavicular joint should be subjected to an open reduction and reconstruction of the acromioclavicular ligament. The final decision is best left to the individual treating orthopedic surgeon, but it is important to make the correct diagnosis and to institute a definitive treatment plan. The author has operated upon far fewer patients with a third-degree acromioclavicular separation in the past 15 years than in the past. Some success has been achieved using a variation of a Kenny–Howard sling to obtain and hold a reduction of the acromioclavicular joint. However, the author obtains the reduction manually and then uses the sling to hold it. If the reduction cannot be obtained, it is advisable not to persist. Simply treat the patient symptomatically, starting his or her rehabilitation when the pain lessens. The disadvantage of using a reduction device is that one has to hold the position for at least 3 weeks and constant readjustments have to be made. If there is no treatment and the clavicle is not reduced and the patient is not doing well, there is always the potential of removing the distal end of the clavicle which should restore normal function without pain.

Fractures of the upper extremity

Fractures of the upper extremity are less common than some soft tissue injuries of the upper extremity and they are less disabling than most fractures of the lower extremity. The common areas for fracture in the upper extremity are the metacarpals (Fig. 12.4), the proximal phalanx of the thumb, the proximal humerus, the

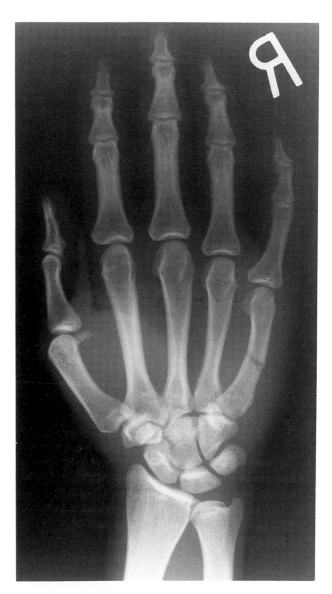

Fig. 12.4 X-ray of a partially displaced fracture of the 5th metacarpal.

distal radius, and the clavicle. Generally the fractures result from falls.

Immediate care

In the vast majority of instances, the racer would recognize that a fracture has occurred because of the instant pain. The acute care on the slope would require protecting the affected body portion by splinting and then getting the skier to a medical facility for a physical and X-rays. The ski patrol person can, by gently palpating the area that is tender, recognize that something is amiss and may be able to make the diagnosis of a fracture. If it is a fracture of one of the metacarpals or phalanges, it is likely that the racer could get down the slopes unaided. However, other fractures such as the clavicle or humerus can be very painful when moved around and movement could cause further damage. The skier would then need assistance in getting down the slopes. Generally, by using a sling and a swathe (wrapping something around the body), the upper extremity can be effectively immobilized. Once in the medical facility, X-rays are taken and in many instances, definitive medical care can be immediately rendered.

Treatment of upper extremity fractures

We will start with the clavicle, the most proximal of the bones affected. Diagnosing a fractured clavicle is easy by both X-ray (Fig. 12.5a) and physical examination. It is unusual to have an open fracture, but displacement of the fracture fragments is common and the fragments are easily seen very close under the skin. Treatment of a fractured clavicle is accomplished by applying a figure-of-eight bandage (Fig. 12.5b) around the torso which will pull the shoulder back and thus bring the fractured distal end of the clavicle into closer approximation to the fractured proximal end. Most clavicular fractures will heal in 6–8 weeks, and although there might be slight displacement of the fragments, usually this is not a problem. The ski competitor should not be on the slopes during that healing time because another fall would result in a refracture of this early healing. Once a fracture has become sticky, usually around 3 weeks, some lower extremity training such as a stationary bicycle could be started. The fracture is solidly healed at about 8 weeks and normal skiing and training can then be resumed.

Fractures of the greater tuberosity of the humerus generally result from a direct blow on the shoulder as the racer falls into the ground. They may occur as a result of a rotator cuff tear which actually pulls away a portion of the greater tuberosity. A greater tuberosity fracture does not cause as much initial pain as a fracture of the clavicle or the humeral shaft, and the racer may feel that he or she has only suffered a bad contusion of the shoulder. Tenderness and inability to abduct the arm properly indicate the necessity of taking an X-ray and a careful look at the area around the greater tuberosity. If such a fracture is undisplaced, it can be treated by putting the arm in a sling for several weeks and starting range of motion exercises within a few days. Healing is usually complete at 6 weeks and by that time, one would expect to have a full range of motion back and full activity could be expected between 6 and 8 weeks. If the fracture fragment is displaced over 5 mm repositioning of that fragment should be done by internal fixation. Once the fracture fragment has been replaced during surgery and held by some internal fixation, range of motion exercises can be initiated after a few days. The healing time is again about 6 weeks and one should wait for that length of time before starting any resistance exercises.

Other fractures of the shoulder or of the humeral shaft are much less common in skiing than they are in certain other sports or in accidents.

Fractures of the distal radius are different in a young ski racer than they are in the older person, when the Colles fracture occurs. In a younger person, displacement is less common and there is less shattering of the bone. The on-the-hill treatment is straightforward with the wrist needing to be protected by a splint and/or a sling while the racer is taken down the hill. X-rays will confirm the diagnosis and definitive treatment can usually be carried out in the ski area facility. Usually, a reduction can be performed with either nerve block anesthesia or, in some instances, by direct infiltration of a block anesthetic into the fracture hematoma. After the reduction is performed, a cast is applied which would usually have to go above the elbow, at least in the early phases.

If the physician is unable to obtain a reduction or to hold a previously gained good position, then a fixation device needs to be used. External fixation has become

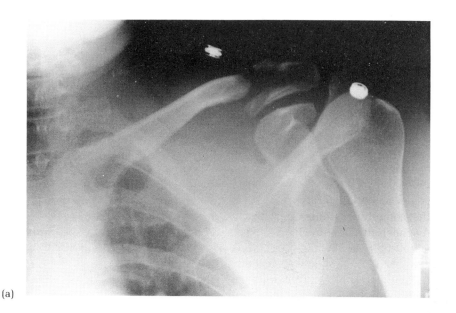

(a)

much more common in the past decade, and either that or a limited open reduction using Kirschner wires may be applicable. The physician should aim for an anatomic reduction, particularly in younger people, and there is usually an excellent chance of obtaining that.

Most distal radius fractures will heal in about 8 weeks, but during that time, finger and shoulder motion must be maintained by doing exercises for the whole upper extremity. Once the fracture is healed, rehabilitation of the upper extremity starts with emphasis placed on motion of the shoulder, wrist and fingers. While strength to the upper extremity is less important than in the lower extremity for ski racing, it is still a vital part for skiing technique. All racers use poles, but the current state-of-the-art in going through slalom poles involving a great deal of contact with the upper extremity and thorax. It may therefore be wise to use some type of protection, such as a plastic splint for a period of time following fracture healing.

Injuries to the hand, particularly to the thumb, are common, and fractures of the proximal phalanx of the thumb or of the metacarpal bones are relatively common. Treatment requires an accurate reduction by longitudinal traction and then the application of an appropriate cast. If it is not possible to obtain an accurate reduction, as shown by post-reduction X-rays, then internal fixation with Kirschner wires may be

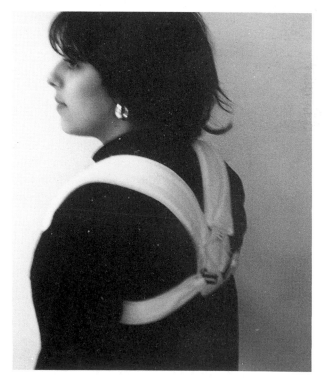

(b)

Fig. 12.5 Fracture of the clavicle: (a) radiogram, and (b) treatment with figure-of-eight bandage.

employed. This would require a hospital setting and expertise in the use of fluoroscopic control while inserting the Kirschner wires. The physician should be particularly careful to note rotation of the fractured phalanx and this can be judged by looking at the distal nail in comparison to the nails of the other fingers.

Most metacarpal and phalangeal fractures heal in 3–4 weeks, when the pins can be taken out and a resumption of normal activity started. One advantage of limited internal fixation with "K" wires is that one is able to get better finger motion in the adjacent fingers because you may only have to use a small splint to hold the fractured bone. As with all upper extremity injuries, particular attention has to be paid to regaining range of motion, or not losing it, in the shoulder, elbow, and other fingers.

An upper extremity fracture is not usually as disabling for the ski racer as a fracture of the lower extremity. However, the ability to use the upper extremities for balance and timing must not be underestimated.

This means that a good range of motion and reasonable muscle strength must return before the skier should resume competition or even practice runs. Emergency care is usually easier for upper extremity injuries simply because the injured skier is able to ambulate and can be transported more easily.

Recommended reading

Carr, D., Johnson, R.J. & Pope, M.H. (1981) Upper extremity injuries in skiing. *Am. J. Sports Med.* **9**:378–383.

Derkask, R., Matyas, J.R., Weaver, J.K. *et al.* (1987) Acute surgical repair of the skier's thumb. *Clin. Orthop. Rel. Res.* **216**:29–33.

Kannus, P. & Johnson, R.J. (1991) Downhill skiing injuries: trends to watch for this season. *J. Musculoskeletal Med.* **8**:13–32.

Johnson, R.J., Ettinger, C.F., Campbell, R.J. & Pope, M.H. (1980) Trends in skiing injuries. *Am. J. Sports Med.* **8(2)**: 106–113.

Chapter 13

Hip

Hip fractures and dislocations are relatively uncommon injuries in modern downhill skiing. Despite their infrequency, the potential for complications following these injuries is high.

Hip fractures are routinely classified by anatomic location. Intracapsular fractures include subcapital (just below the femoral head) and transcervical (along the femoral neck). Since this distinction does not change the method of treatment of these injuries, in this chapter the term intracapsular fracture will encompass both types. These fractures result in a higher rate of nonunion and avascular necrosis than do extracapsular fractures. Intracapsular hip fractures may be further subdivided into nondisplaced and displaced fracture categories. A displaced fracture leads to immediate cessation of blood flow to the femoral head when it is intracapsular. Loss of blood flow to the femoral head may lead to poor healing and subsequent necrosis of the femoral head with or without secondary collapse and incongruity.

Extracapsular fractures of the hip are more commonly termed intertrochanteric fractures. They occur in the bone between the greater and lesser trochanter and because the blood supply remains intact the potential for healing is better that with intracapsular fractures. They are frequently the result of great violence and marked comminution of the fracture is common.

Dislocation of the hip is commonly classified by the location of the femoral head with reference to the acetabulum. Anterior dislocations are much less common that posterior dislocations. There may or may not be an attendant femoral head and/or acetabular fracture. Even less common is the central hip dislocation in which the head is pushed through the medial wall of the acetabulum with fracture of one or both.

Injury recognition

It is imperative that ski patrol personnel are familiar with the clinical presentation of a hip injury so that appropriate steps may be taken immediately on the mountain to ensure the skier the best possible long-term result. The first step is the ability to recognize these injuries based upon limb position. Displaced intracapsular fractures usually present with some shortening, abduction and external rotation of the involved limb (Fig. 13.1). On the other hand, displaced intertrochanteric fractures usually result in more extensive shortening and external rotation (up to 90°). In anterior hip dislocations, the limb is often in a "position of immodesty," implying that the thigh is in a position of more extreme abduction and external

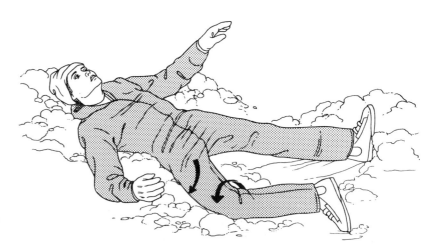

Fig. 13.1 A significantly shortened externally rotated right lower limb suggestive of a displaced intracapsular hip fracture.

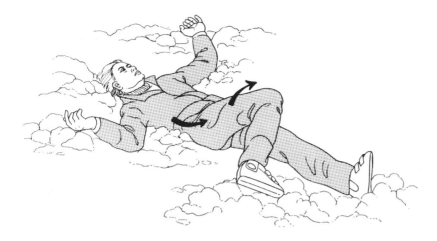

Fig. 13.2 Adduction/internal rotation of the hip suggestive of a posterior hip dislocation.

rotation. Posterior dislocations, usually present with the hip positioned in slight flexion, adduction, and internal rotation (Fig. 13.2).

Another useful source of information is the location of pain reported by the patient prior to being moved. Pain in the upper thigh, groin, or trochanteric area is characteristic. Gentle palpation to elicit the area of maximal tenderness may direct the observer to the location of injury. One should assess and record the mechanism of injury, and pay special attention to snow conditions, type of run, fall versus collision, skier position during fall and condition of ski/binding complex. This information can be useful not only in making a presumptive diagnosis, but also in assisting with injury analysis and prevention in the future for other skiers.

Immediate care

Immediate care for the injured skier should follow the basic guidelines for acute care of the injured athlete. A rapid assessment of injuries should be made by qualified ski patrol personnel starting with the respiratory system, followed by the cardiovascular system, neurological system, and finally the musculoskeletal system. Breathing rate (normal 10–30 times/min) and pattern should be observed. If either of these is abnormal, quickly check, and if necessary, clear the airway. The chest should also be observed for unstable rib segments (flail) or sucking wounds. The cardiovascular system can be appraised quickly and simply for overall function by checking for a radial or carotid pulse (rate and character) and for bleeding sites. In the event that a pulse is not present, cardiopulmonary resuscitation (CPR) should be immediately instituted and a medical team alerted by radio. Sterile compressive dressings should be applied to bleeding sites. A quick evaluation of neurological status should be made starting with level of consciousness, progressing to the presence of gross motor function in all four extremities. Any gross neurological abnormality or complaint of neck and/or back pain should warrant extreme care in moving the patient to prevent further neurological injury.

The musculoskeletal system should be inspected grossly for areas of pain/tenderness and deformity/limb position. With specific evidence of a hip injury, especially a fracture, a splint should be applied prior to transfer unless CPR or other life-sustaining maneuvers take precedence. Only gentle traction should be applied to the limb in an attempt to align the extremity anatomically. The Thomas splint is a traction device that can maintain limb position most effectively for hip fractures as it rests proximally on the ischial tuberosity and it applies gentle traction through the straps at the ankle (Fig. 13.3). This splint is available to most ski patrols, but it should be noted that it requires two personnel for application. If this condition is not met, or the Thomas splint is not available, then the limb can be braced during transport with pillows or blankets to decrease motion at the injury site. When limb position suggests dislocation, the traction splint should not be used.

After the patient's injury has been adequately sta-

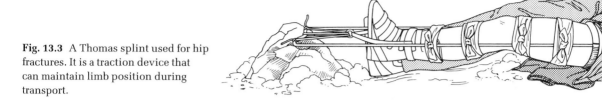

Fig. 13.3 A Thomas splint used for hip fractures. It is a traction device that can maintain limb position during transport.

bilized, the most efficacious method of conveying the patient to an emergency care facility should be instituted. It is imperative that involved personnel on the mountain assure that the patient receives nothing by mouth (NPO) in the event that definitive treatment might require emergency surgical treatment. Emergency room care of a skier with a suspected hip fracture or dislocation should begin with a complete systematic reassessment. The injured hip should be radiographed with an anteroposterior pelvic view, anteroposterior hip view, and cross-table lateral view. Following this evaluation, orthopedic consultation should be obtained.

Treatment

The orthopedist confronted with a hip fracture or dislocation in the skier should keep in mind that the injury requires accurate assessment and rapid care to optimize the final result. Anatomic reduction and stable fixation must be obtained to facilitate reha-

bilitation and regain function in this highly active patient population. Specifically, for intracapsular femoral neck fractures which are impacted or non-displaced, rigid internal fixation with multiple screws (three in most cases is sufficient) usually provides the greatest success (Figs 13.4 & 13.5). For displaced fractures which require open reduction, anatomic alignment and fixation should be performed through a Watson–Jones approach. Bone grafting for posterior comminution should be performed if necessary, and fixation gained with multiple screws. It is of utmost importance that the displaced intracapsular hip fracture be treated urgently in order to preserve or restore femoral head blood flow.

Most fractures of the hip will occur in younger people who are racing as opposed to an older population. Some older skiers will race in the senior division, but fractures occurring in this group will probably be treated the same way as in a younger group. Experienced senior ski racers are likely to have good bone stock and joint surfaces, thus replacement pros-

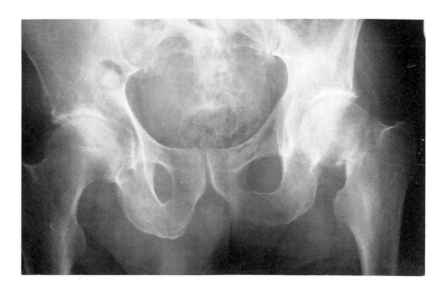

Fig. 13.4 X-ray of intracapsular hip fracture.

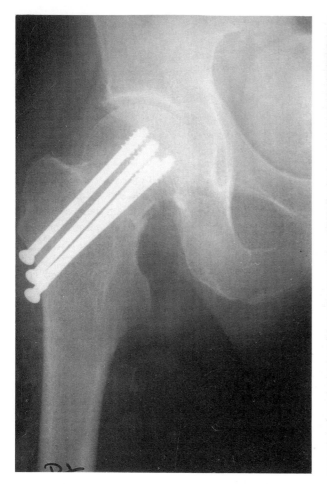

Fig. 13.5 X-ray showing rigid internal fixation with multiple screws. A procedure used for intracapsular femoral neck fractures.

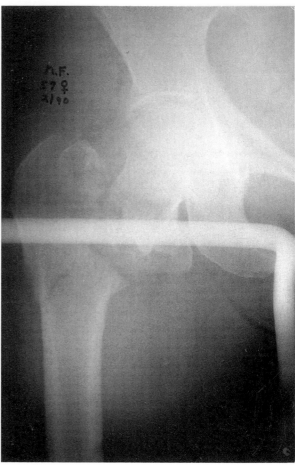

Fig. 13.6 X-ray showing intertrochanteric femur fracture.

thetics are less likely in this population group than in the older nonskiing population.

Since intertrochanteric hip fractures are extracapsular, they are less likely to result in disruption of femoral head blood flow. The lack of disruption of flow to the femoral head in turn makes surgical treatment an urgent, not an emergent, procedure. Anatomic reduction to maintain normal hip geometry and length is essential if a normal functioning hip is to be obtained (Figs 13.6 & 13.7). The standard type of fixation is a sliding nail-plate device. Maximum posterior and medial bony contact is essential for fracture stability. Hip dislocations may be reduced either in the emergency room with the patient under sedative or analgesic medication, or in the operating room under general anesthesia. One gentle closed attempt should be made, and if unsuccessful, an open reduction performed. Radiographic examination should document the congruency of the reduction. If incongruency is present, a computerized tomography scan should be performed to look for loose fragments in the joint that might preclude complete reduction. If fragments are present, they should be removed surgically.

Rehabilitation

Maximum rehabilitation from hip injury in the skier requires complete cooperation and open communi-

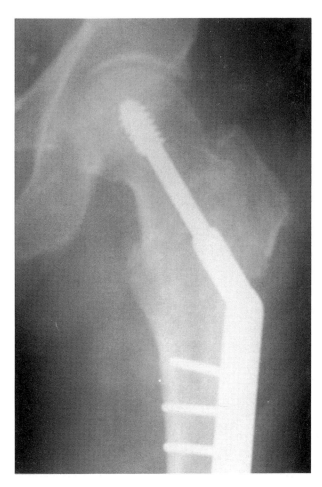

Fig. 13.7 X-ray showing a sliding nail plate device, a standard type of fixation for displaced intertrochanteric femur fractures.

and regain hip mobility. Following this, a program is started of strengthening certain muscles, but it is important to try and decrease the effect of hip joint loading from muscle contraction. Examples are unresisted ankle plantar flexion, dorsiflexion, inversion/eversion, and quadriceps/hamstring set exercises without straight leg raising. Well-leg bicycling can be performed with the operated limb resting on a stool as soon as the patient is comfortable sitting on the bicycle. The patient may find it beneficial to remove the pedal on the operated side to facilitate this procedure. During the early rehabilitation period, a deep-water unweighted resisted training program using a flotation device may be performed. In this way, aerobic conditioning as well as gentle strengthening of muscles around the hip joint may be safely performed. Once fracture union can be documented radiographically, usually 6–9 months postoperatively, the patient may begin a more sport-specific program aimed at functional training. The use of an elastic resistance cord for ski-specific muscle strengthening and coordination may be initiated. The patient may thus work on ski-specific motions such as side-to-side mobility and balance. The elastic cord is also useful to train both concentrically and eccentrically, which more closely simulates skiing than other exercise regimens.

Extracapsular hip fractures, on the other hand, are inherently more stable provided there is medial bony contact obtained during reduction. Hence, stability is more easily maintained with internal fixation. Therefore, more aggressive early weight bearing may be acceptable. If appropriate, partial weight bearing with crutches should be encouraged as soon as the patient is comfortable. A gentle passive range of motion program should be instituted early along with strengthening of muscle groups around the hip. A deep-water program is beneficial in these cases to allow comfortable early resistive training of the operated limb. Well-leg cycling should be started immediately after surgery, and unlike intracapsular fractures, the operated limb may be cycled as early as 2 weeks postoperatively. As soon as radiographs show callus and the patient is comfortable with full weight bearing, resistive training with the elastic resistance cord may be initiated. In the presence of full radiographic healing, it is possible for sport-specific training to begin. Return to skiing may be anticipated as soon as 9 months after the injury.

cation among the orthopedist, trainer/therapist, and patient. The rehabilitation program must take into account the injury type, acute treatment, stage of healing of bone and soft tissues, and patient motivation. For intracapsular fractures, strength of the internal fixation is more critical than with extracapsular fractures because minimal stability is imparted by the bony anatomy. Therefore, it is recommended that only partial weight bearing (toe touch) be allowed for 6–8 weeks, followed by a gradual progression to full weight bearing. However, numerous techniques can be used prior to full weight bearing to rehabilitate patients. The protocol should begin with gentle range of motion exercises to maintain motion of other joints

Following reduction of a hip dislocation, the patient should be maintained in 2.25–3 kg (5–7 lb) of skin traction until the acute pain of injury subsides. Early aggressive active and passive range of motion exercises should be instituted within the stable range of motion as determined immediately after reduction. Once the patient is comfortable, partial weight bearing should be started with gradual progression to full weight bearing as tolerated. Femoral head and/or acetabular fractures should be treated with altered weight bearing, determined by the specific injury patterns.

It should be emphasized that while protecting the healing hip, the patient's aerobic conditioning should be maintained. Depending upon the hip stability pattern, a deep-water program may be instituted to allow gentle unweighted resistive training of the injured and uninjured limbs. Once soft tissue healing around the hip has occurred, a more aggressive rehabilitation program involving cycling of the injured limb and light stretch cord resistive training may be begun. Prior to resumption of heavy resistive and sport-specific training, a bone scan may be advisable to assure vascularity of the femoral head. If an avascular head is detected, aggressive exercises should be delayed indefinitely to decrease the possibility of late segmental collapse of the femoral head. At present, there is no consensus regarding specific treatment for this complication.

Prior to resumption of downhill skiing, patients in all injury categories should undergo a sport-specific test of conditioning. The test allows a more accurate assessment of patient's adequacy of rehabilitation prior to loading the joint fully during sport.

Risk factors

The overall incidence of hip fracture or dislocation in the downhill skier is low, and so is the availability of well-documented demographic data regarding associated risk factors. Therefore, one might choose to look at the factors associated with lower extremity ski injuries in general. Most injuries occurred during falls, and approximately 20% occurred during collisions in two studies (Fig. 13.8). Collisions accounted for one-third of all femoral fractures (both shaft and hip) in a study by Yvars. In this study, causes of injury in the noncollision group (falls) were skiing at high

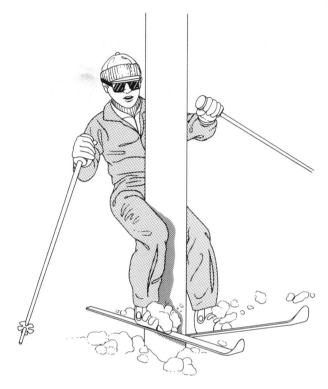

Fig. 13.8 A skier sustaining injuries due to collision.

speeds, loss of control, and icy slopes. Most collisions and out of control falls were in the age group under 30 years. Beginning skiers were noted in one study to have a three times greater risk of injury than more experienced skiers. However, no correlation to injury type was made. Moreover, in another review, beginning skiers who had formal instruction had a lower injury rate than those who did not receive training.

Increasing age correlated with a higher incidence of hip fractures in a small series of femur fractures, suggesting a higher risk of hip fractures in patients over 40. Three out of the four hip fractures were in patients over 60 years of age. The apparent increased incidence of hip fractures associated with skiing in patients this age would correlate with the decreased bone mass that is expected with aging.

Finally, newer equipment, particularly bindings, has decreased the incidence of injury of the lower extremity. Whether there is a relationship between binding quality and adjustment as they relate to hip injury is still unclear. However, binding safety unquestionably must be emphasized in any overall injury prevention program.

Prevention of injuries

While no consensus exists concerning risk factors for hip fracture or dislocation, certain injury avoidance measures can be recommended. Skier education is paramount. It should consist of formal beginner instruction on skiing techniques along with public awareness programs for the more experienced skiers on skiing safety, training techniques and equipment updates. Annual binding adjustments should be routine for skiers who own skis.

Return to sport

Ultimately, the goal of health-care professionals involved in care of skiers who sustain hip fractures, is to return the athlete to downhill skiing. The timing of return is complex and relies on both the presence of fracture union and adequate conditioning. Most hip fractures will require a period of at least 9 months to heal adequately before safe resumption of skiing.

Higher level skiers may find that internal fixation devices used for fracture treatment cause enough symptoms to warrant their removal. Controversy exists as to the amount of time a patient should avoid high-stress activity following hardware removal. Specific activity avoidance decreases the likelihood of fracture through screw holes which remain as stress risers. The AO (Association for Osteosynthesis) group recommends that no extreme levels of athletic activities be performed for at least 4 months after metal removal. However, refracture may occur as late as 2 years after metal extraction. Finally, older recreational skiers with osteopenic bone should be advised to alter their sporting activities to a level less strenuous than downhill skiing or at a minimum, choose the safest terrain and skiing conditions.

Recommended reading

DeLee, J.C. (1984) Fractures and dislocations of the hip in adults. In Rockwood, C.A. & Green, P.D. (eds) *Fractures in Adults*. Philadelphia: J.B. Lippincott, pp. 1211–1356.

Epstein, H.C. (1980) *Traumatic Dislocation of the Hip*. Baltimore: Williams & Wilkins.

Tapper, E.M. (1978) Ski injuries from 1939 to 1976: the Sun Valley experience. *Am. J. Sports Med.* **6(3)**:114–121.

Chapter 14
Femur

Injury incidence

Femoral fractures are rare in Alpine skiing, and there has not been a large reported series of this particular ski injury. Yvars reported on 23 ski-related femoral fractures which occurred during an 8-year period, and Tapper reported 11 femoral fractures out of 4227 ski-related injuries. O'Malley reported on 115 cases of femoral fractures collected over an 18-year period, and the combined incidence of femoral fractures in these series was approximately one per 100 000 skier days.

A number of risk factors have been identified with regard to skiing injuries. However, few have been found that directly impact the incidence of femoral fractures. Hauser reported a relatively high risk for lower extremity equipment-related (LEER) injuries in beginning skiers and children and attributed this increased risk to poor equipment and incorrect binding settings. The majority of injuries in this LEER category include severe ligamentous injuries to the knee and fractures of the tibia. Injuries in expert skiers usually were not equipment related and were primarily due to high-speed skiing permitted by improved equipment and improved trail grooming. It has been noted that the higher the speed of the skier prior to the accident, the higher in the body the injury occurred and hence, there is a greater potential for femoral fractures versus lower leg injuries in the high-speed skier, such as a ski racer.

Ekeland reported that skiing ability and experience had a statistically significant effect on injury rate and that beginners had an injury ratio approximately four times higher than the average in his studies. Those skiers with previous formal instruction had significantly fewer injuries compared with the group which had no formal instruction. Also of note was that skiers aged 15–19 were significantly more prone to injuries than skiers in all other age groups.

Data published by Hauser, Ekeland, and Lystad all concurred that poor bindings were a common cause of injury in both inexperienced skiers and those under the age of 10. However, bindings did not affect the frequency of femoral fractures. Yvars reported an increase in ski-related femoral injuries during the last 3 years of his study. He felt that this increase in femoral fractures was due to high-speed cruising which was invited by well-groomed slopes and perhaps by longer, more stable skis. He stated that high-speed skiing requires strength, skill, judgment, and alertness to maintain course and control, and that in the younger skier, prudence may not be held with much reverence and a casual attitude towards skiing may be one factor responsible for the increase in femoral fractures in this particular group.

Injury recognition

Femoral fractures are caused by extreme forces (Fig. 14.1) and may result in other bodily injuries other than to the femur. A systematic approach should be taken in the event of such an injury. Proper care consists of the recognition and treatment at the injury site, followed by transport to an appropriate facility where definitive fracture stabilization can be performed.

Proper assessment of the injured skier begins with the first impression formed by the rescuer as he or she approaches the injury site. Upon reaching the skier, a first impression should already be formed and the primary survey can then begin. This primary survey includes identification of life-threatening emergencies and an assessment of the status of the respiratory and circulatory systems, the patient's responsiveness, and any severe bleeding. The mechanism of injury must be taken into account at that time as well as the possibility of imminent danger to the injured skier and ever the rescuer. In the case of a femoral fracture, the skier may be in close proximity to a pole, tree, life tower, etc., since the majority of these injuries are caused by collisions. After the primary survey is completed, a secondary survey should examine the remaining organ systems and look at the other extremities.

Following that, attention is paid to the obviously injured thigh, which in the case of a femoral fracture,

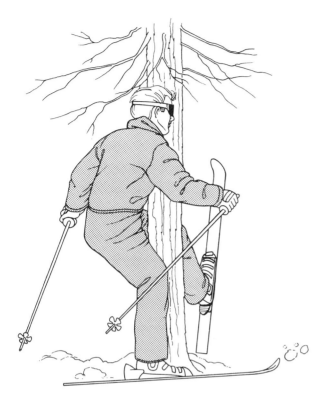

Fig. 14.1 A skier colliding with a fixed object such as a tree is the most common mechanism which causes a femur fracture.

may well show malposition of the fracture fragments. The patient would probably be complaining of pain in the thigh and even a cursory palpation may reveal crepitus, limb deformity, and may cause excruciating pain. Gross swelling of the area may not be noticeable, if the clothing is bulky, but remember that a fracture of the femur can cause 1–2 l of blood loss within the soft tissues. Shortening of the thigh relative to the other leg may be noted due to fracture fragment overriding. There may be a knee effusion present if there is a fracture of the distal femur which communicates with the joint or it may be due to concomitant trauma to the knee joint with a blow against a fixed object. The presence of torn or blood-soaked clothing over the fracture site suggests an open fracture and hence, a more severe injury.

Immediate care

After the patient's cardiovascular and respiratory systems have been stabilized as much as possible and any other injuries have been addressed, attention is directed to the femoral fracture. One may elect to perform a gross reduction of the fracture to achieve some anatomic alignment and to enable the fracture to be more easily stabilized with a traction splint or rigid fixation splint. This must be done so that the injured skier can then be transported down the hill for further treatment. In the case of a femoral fracture, it is probably best to remove the patient off the hill and quickly on the way to a medical facility where adequate assessment of the fracture can be performed and treatment started. There is some urgency to this. It is probably best to bypass the local ski medical facility and get the patient on the way to hospital for definitive treatment.

Treatment

Early treatment of femoral fractures begins with accurate recognition and classification of the fracture. Treatment varies depending on type and location of the fracture. Open fractures require early irrigation and debridement followed by appropriate definitive therapy. Treatment of closed fractures may be delayed if necessary; however, recent reports have shown better results if the fracture is rigidly stabilized early.

Femur fractures can be subdivided by anatomic location into intracapsular hip fractures, extracapsular hip fractures, subtrochanteric, shaft, and supracondylar fractures. Intra- and extracapsular hip fractures will be discussed in another chapter. In this chapter, we will consider subtrochanteric, femoral shaft, and supracondylar fractures.

Subtrochanteric fractures

Subtrochanteric femur fractures are defined as those fractures which occur between the lesser trochanter and a point 5 cm distal. They account for 15% of all fractures at the proximal femur. These injuries may be further subdivided based on the level, configuration, and number of fracture fragments.

Transport of a subtrochanteric fracture requires knowledge of the injury and deforming muscle forces. Due to the location of the fracture, the psoas muscle flexes the proximal fragment making hip extension painful. In these cases, the leg is stabilized with the hip and knee flexed. At times, the patient may be most comfortable in a sitting position. Once the skier reaches the hospital emergency room, definitive treatment can be commenced.

Treatment of subtrochanteric fractures varies according to classification, inherent stability, and degree of comminution. In fractures with inordinate amounts of comminution, traction may be the first line of treatment due to inability to provide rigid fixation. If the degree of comminution does not obviate internal fixation, a number of methods are available. The Zickel nail is the device with the most extensive track record. This is an intramedullary device with a flanged nail placed into the femoral neck for proximal stability and a stem placed into the canal for distal stability. Union rates of 90% have been reported with the use of this device. Complications with use of the Zickel nail include the risk of refracture after removal of the nail especially when used in younger patients. Nonunion rates of 5% have also been reported.

Use of sliding hip screws with long side plates has been advocated by the AO/ASIF (Association for Osteosynthesis/Association for the Study of the Problems of Internal Fixation) group. Union rates have been reported as high as 95%. These devices provide rigid fixation and allow early motion; however, care must be taken to ensure adequate medial support with the use of bone grafting, if necessary, to improve success rates. If medial support is not established, nonunion may result with ensuing hardware failure. If the lesser trochanter is intact, a standard interlocking femoral nail can be used to provide both proximal and distal stability.

For open subtrochanteric fractures, surgical options include traction or external fixation, either as a means of definitive treatment or as primary treatment prior to delayed internal fixation.

Femoral shaft fractures

Femoral shaft fractures can be classified based on fracture configuration or degree of comminution. It is the degree of comminution and location of the fracture that most influences the method of treatment chosen.

Proper transport of a patient with a femoral shaft fracture begins with gross realignment followed by placement in a traction splint. The most commonly used traction splint is the Thomas splint (Fig. 14.2). Other commercially available traction splints include Hare and Sager splints, and the Kendrick traction device. If a commercially manufactured splint is not available, one can be made with a single ski or two ski pole technique. These devices are used to prevent overriding of bone fragments and to decrease limb shortening, pain, and bleeding. The skier can then be transported to a proper facility for definitive care including palpation of pulses, examination of wounds, and radiographic examination.

At the present time, the standard of care for treatment of femoral shaft fractures is reamed intramedullary nailing with or without locking screws, based on the fracture pattern and location (Figs 14.3 & 14.4). Those fractures with inherent stability and little comminution which occur in the isthmus of the femur may not require locking. Fractures with significant

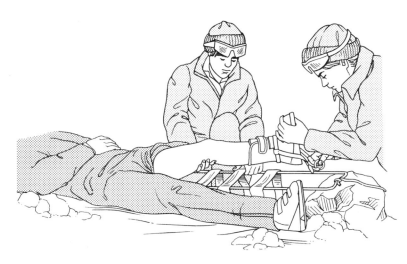

Fig. 14.2 A femur fracture should be stabilized on the mountain in a mobile traction splint such as a Thomas splint. The skier can then safely be transported down the hill.

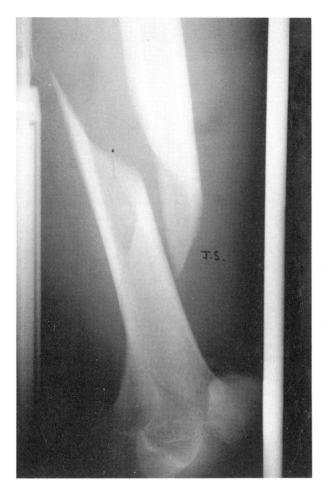

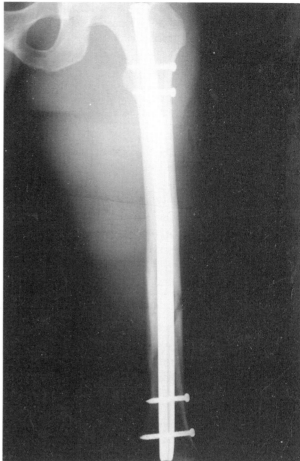

Fig. 14.3 A typical mid-shaft femur fracture caused by a ski accident.

Fig. 14.4 Standard care for closed femoral shaft fractures is intramedullary nailing.

comminution and those located in the proximal or distal third of the femur often require locking at one or both ends. This method can be employed in almost all fractures of the shaft of the femur with the exception of Gustillo grade III open fractures and those fractures which extend into the joint, either proximally or distally. This method can help to assure proper length and rotation, and it allows the patient early motion to begin rehabilitation. Studies have shown that early mobilization after rigid fixation of a femur fracture speeds recovery and avoids systemic complications.

Infection rates with intramedullary nailing have been reported from 0.5 to 1.5% for closed fractures and from 0 to 4% for open fractures. The most frequent complication is malunion, but locked nailing tech-niques have decreased this problem in recent years. Nonunion and delayed union occur relatively in-frequently with the use of reamed intramedullary nailing.

Femoral shaft fractures may also be plated, but this technique is usually reserved for situations in which there are ipsilateral femoral shaft and neck fractures or in those patients with concomitant arterial injury. One complication of compression plating is a higher than normal infection rate compared to other operative treatments. Another complication is stress shielding of the bone directly under the plate. The ensuing loss of bone may lead to hardware failure, refracture, non-union, or delayed union.

Open femoral fractures may be treated with reamed

intramedullary nailing if soft tissue damage is not too extensive. If, however, there is extensive soft tissue stripping and muscle damage, external fixation may be preferable.

Supracondylar fractures

Supracondylar fractures can be the most disabling femoral fractures, especially if there is a displaced intra-articular component. Of the various fracture classifications described, especially useful is the AO/ASIF system which considers rotation, comminution, and the intra-articular nature of the fracture. Fractures which cause severe joint disruption have a guarded prognosis due to the high incidence of post-traumatic degenerative arthritis.

If a supracondylar fracture is suspected at the time of initial examination, assessment should include careful inspection of distal pulses and neurologic status. The neurovascular bundle in the popliteal fossa may be damaged by jagged bone ends of supracondylar fractures.

Care and transport involve gentle alignment of the extremity followed by placement in a lower extremity fixation splint. Traction splints should not be used due to the possibility of causing further nerve or vessel damage. The patient should be transported quickly off the hill so neurovascular status can be more closely monitored and definitive treatment can be started.

Supracondylar fractures without intra-articular involvement and some nondisplaced intra-articular fractures may be treated with nonoperative immobilization, provided that anatomic alignment can be maintained. Displaced supracondylar–intercondylar fractures are best treated with open reduction and internal fixation.

Current standards of care for supracondylar–intercondylar fractures involve the use of angled blade plates or condylar compression screws. Both methods allow rigid fixation of the articular surface under direct vision to restore precisely the anatomy of the joint. Long side plates are attached, and early protected range of motion can begin soon after surgery. Complications encountered with the use of internal fixation include infection, nonunion, malunion, and late degenerative arthritis. Complications of fixation with flexible rods are similar, however, indications for use of these devices are fewer.

Open supracondylar femur fractures may require external fixation as definitive treatment or as a means of primary treatment prior to delayed internal fixation. Complications of external fixation include pin tract infection, delayed union, malalignment, and loss of joint motion.

Rehabilitation

Rehabilitation following femur fractures and other lower extremity injuries can be divided into three categories: (i) psychologic, (ii) physiologic, and (iii) physical rehabilitation. Psychologic rehabilitation begins with the formation of realistic goals for the patient and can help to maintain appropriate self image and alleviate the frustration of weeks of immobility which can occur after injury.

Physiologic rehabilitation is designed to maintain pre-injury aerobic fitness and can be commenced as early as the first postoperative day. It has been reported that maintenance of aerobic fitness by cross-education training utilizing an aerobic or physiologic conditioning program can benefit the patient by providing an immediate sense of psychologic well being. This type of early postoperative training avoids the loss of aerobic conditioning which can occur as early as 6–8 weeks after immobility.

After a femur fracture, aerobic conditioning can be commenced well before osseous union is apparent and can be accomplished by well-leg or both-leg stationary cycling, or through use of deep-water therapy assisted by a flotation device. Following osseous union, more aggressive aerobic training should include activities such as use of a surgical tubing resistance routine or by jogging, uphill running, or playing soccer or racquet sports.

Maintenance of upper extremity conditioning can be commenced on the day of surgery and can be continued thereafter. It is the muscles of the torso and arms which maintain the balance of the skier and help avoid falls. In the competitive skier, it is important to begin exercising uninjured extremities as soon as possible to maintain pre-injury levels of fitness.

Physical rehabilitation of the fractured femur may begin on the first postoperative day with maintenance of knee and hip range of motion in the injured extremity. Early passive range of motion is of primary importance for femoral shaft and supracondylar fractures to prevent muscular and intra-articular adhesions. This early motion may be accomplished with a continuous passive motion (CPM) machine, or intermittently with manual assistance. Vigorous active range of motion of the knee may begin when the patient can perform unassisted straight leg raises.

After rigid intramedullary stabilization or bone plate application, full hip and knee motion can be performed without external bracing; however, after Zickel nailing or flexible intramedullary nailing, protective bracing may be necessary. As fracture healing progresses, the patient should continue to perform straight-leg exercises and ankle pumps to maintain thigh and calf strength.

Early weight bearing may be commenced as soon as pain allows in rigidly fixed, stable fracture configurations. In other less stable fractures, weight bearing may be started when radiographic evidence of bridging callus develops. Femoral fractures can be expected to heal within 16–20 weeks, and the skier may commence more aggressive training subsequent to radiographic evidence of complete osseous union, absence of pain, and return of strength to the muscles of the involved leg.

After osseous healing occurs, specific muscle groups should be reconditioned in order to return the skier to the slopes more efficiently. The quadriceps is one of the most important muscle groups to consider in rehabilitation and strength training after a femur fracture. It is through the use of these muscles that the patient maintains his or her position in space. In reconditioning, both eccentric and concentric contractions must be stressed since these muscles contract in both modes during skiing. Concentric exercises can be accomplished through the use of straight-leg raises and knee extensions, but any arc of motion which causes patellofemoral pain must be avoided. Eccentric contractions can be produced through the use of a stretch cord program or progressive free weight program.

The hamstrings should not be neglected in the reconditioning exercise program. These muscles are used for both initiation and completion of turns, and they oppose the anterior subluxing force of the quadriceps mechanism. Good tone in this muscle group can help prevent further knee injury.

Once complete osseous healing has occurred, and strength, range of motion, and endurance are regained, the final phase of rehabilitation begins. It is at this point in the rehabilitation program that ski-specific exercises are started, including side-to-side hops, jumping rope, one-third knee bends, or use of a side-to-side slide board. These exercises can be coupled with a surgical tubing resistance program and incorporated into specific ski motions which provide both eccentric and concentric contractions of the involved muscle groups. These exercises should be incorporated into endurance training, preparing the patient for return to skiing. This return will usually be 9–12 months following a femoral shaft fracture for the competitive skier.

Prevention of injuries

Avoidance of femoral fractures on the ski slopes should start with proper muscle conditioning and training in order to maintain course and control on the slopes. Training should be augmented by formal instruction for the inexperienced skier. Equipment should be well maintained and all skiers, both recreational and competitive, should be cognizant of the fact that high speeds, which are generated on the slopes due to new technologies now available in equipment and slope grooming, are likely to lead to more severe injuries.

Conclusion

Femur fractures are rare but can cause severe disability. Risk factors for femur fracture include young age, inexperience, and high-speed skiing. Formal instruction and careful regard for the dangers of high-speed skiing may decrease the risk of femur fracture. Three types of femur fractures have been discussed: subtrochanteric, femoral shaft, and supracondylar femur fractures. Treatment differs for each fracture. Rehabilitation hinges on setting early goals, maintaining range of motion and aerobic conditioning, and regaining strength after osseous union.

If proper recognition, treatment, and rehabilitation are employed, the skier with a femur fracture may be able to return to the slopes within 9–12 months after injury.

Recommended reading

Bowman, W.D. (1988) *The National Ski Patrol's Outdoor Emergency Care System.* Lakewood, Colorado: The National Ski Patrol System Inc.

Chapman, M.A. (1986) The role of intramedullary fixation in open fractures. *Clin. Orthop.* **212**:26.

Johnson, R.F., Ettlinger, C.F. & Shealy, J.E. (1987) Ski injury trends. In Mote, C.D. & Johnson, R.J. (eds) *Skiing Trauma and Safety: 7th International Symposium ASTM Special Publication.* Philadelphia: ASTM.

Steadman, J.R. (1982) Rehabilitation of skiing injuries. *Clin. Sports Med.* **1**:289.

Yvars, M.D. & Kanner, H.R. (1984) Ski fractures of the femur. *Am. J. Sports Med.* **12**:386.

Chapter 15

Knee

Knee injuries from Alpine skiing have remained relatively constant since statistics have been kept; however, the distribution of injuries has changed significantly. The incidence of medial collateral ligament (MCL) injuries of the knee, which are usually due to abduction and external rotation of the lower leg, have decreased, while the likelihood of anterior cruciate ligament (ACL) injury has increased dramatically. The reasons for the change would seem to include several factors which have occurred during the last 30 years.

Injury incidence

Equipment

First, there has been a dramatic change in equipment. The boots are higher and stiffer, particularly in the rear (Fig. 15.1). This design creates a fulcrum which places a direct forward pressure on the ACL and its secondary restraints. This fulcrum is particularly significant during backward falls where the skier's center of gravity is falling back while the ski and boot are moving forward. This creates forward displacement on the upper tibia in relationship to the femur, placing the cruciate at risk. Additional biomechanical forces at work during this type of fall include extension of the upper body which relaxes the hamstring, flexion of the knee which does the same, quadriceps contraction which creates an anterior drawer effect on the cruciate, and slight degrees of rotation of the tibia which make the cruciate taut.

Other factors which have been implicated are the reversing of the camber of the ski which tends to jet it forward, and the compression of the heel and toe pieces which occurs with this reverse camber.

Favorable factors in diminishing the ACL deformation may be upward toe release in some bindings, although no statistical proof is available.

Technique

There have been technique changes which may affect knee biomechanics. As a skier progresses from stem turns toward parallel turns with increased acceleration through the turn, the cruciate may become more at risk. This could explain the extremely high incidence of cruciate tears in competitive skiers. Other factors which are important in ski injuries include conditioning and terrain.

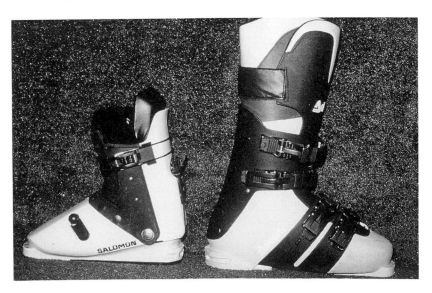

Fig. 15.1 A high ski boot compared to a low ski boot.

Conditioning

The possibility that fatigue may be a factor in injuries has been suggested. As the quadriceps becomes fatigued, it loses power. This loss of power could create an inability to recover from injury-producing falls. As a result, conditioning programs are encouraged which involve endurance, long-term concentric and eccentric training, and general agility.

Terrain

With better slope grooming, the skier can progress to more advanced terrain without achieving the necessary level of skill which is commensurate with the increased difficulty in maintaining control. The potential for injury due to obstacles, including trees, towers, and other skiers is accordingly enhanced. Control problems resulting from high speed on steep slopes is an additional factor which increases the risk of injury.

The multitude of factors in this area makes statistics difficult to obtain, but skiers should take special care when skiing in an area where their skill does not match the difficulty of the terrain.

Seasonal variation

Alpine competitive skiing training is ideally divided into two seasons. The first consists of dry land training which is designed to create a sound aerobic base for the athlete. Agility, specific muscle fiber-type training, endurance training, and training for the repetitive up-and-down motions (concentric and eccentric contraction) involved in skiing are also addressed. The second season is the on-snow training, supplemented with a continuation of sport-specific dry land training. This combination of activities is important to all skiers, not just competitive skiers.

Each of these periods has specific injury possibilities; and will be considered separately.

Dry land training injuries

Injuries associated with dry land training are usually caused by overstress (Fig. 15.2). The choice of sports during the period can have a major effect on the types of injury. For instance, if cycling and elastic resistance training are employed, the chances of injury other than overstress are diminished. If soccer is added, the risk of ankle and knee injury is materially increased. If motor-cross is added, the risk of serious injury is increased as well. One of the specific activities which correlates extremely well with skiing is downhill running, but it enhances the tendency for patello-femoral problems. Racquet sports also correlate well with skiing, but they present a multitude of associated injury possibilities. Weight training involving elastic resistance, machines or free weights has inherent

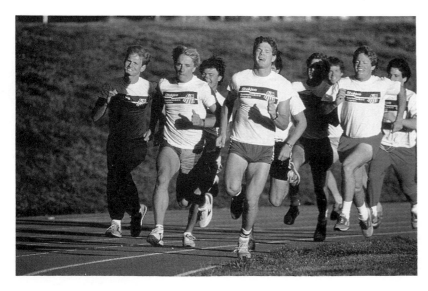

Fig. 15.2 A skier performing interval training. Types of injuries sustained during dry land training are influenced by the choice of sports other than skiing performed during that period.

injuries which should be anticipated and avoided. Thus, the choice of activity can materially affect the likelihood of dry land injury.

General anterior knee pain

Overstress injuries sustained in dry land ski training usually involve the patellofemoral joint. These injuries can affect the patella, trochlear groove of the femur, plica synovialis, fat pad, or the quadriceps or patellar tendon. Of these areas, we have placed particular emphasis on the plica in skiing. The repetitive up-and-down motion required in skiing creates significant stress on these areas and increases stiffness and potential for anterior knee pain. Fat pad impingement, chondromalacia, and tendinitis are common primary or secondary sequelae.

The pathologic nature of these tissues has been proven anecdotally by response to treatment of numerous competitive skiers from several countries. We have statistically documented this same phenomena in our practice.

The initial treatment for all these anterior knee pain problems is essentially the same during the nonoperative period. However, surgical treatments vary, and each will be discussed separately.

Nonoperative treatment

Many conditions cause anterior knee pain and the operative treatment for these conditions is similar. Treatment is divided into two stages.

First, an initial evaluation of the problem is done and the diagnosis made. The diagnosis may include chondromalacia, plica syndrome, or tendinitis. The approach to each problem includes rest of the injured area combined with strengthening of the surrounding muscle groups. This can be accomplished by careful evaluation of the response of the painful area to various forms of exercise, eliminating exercises or parts of range of motion during a specific exercise which cause pain.

Exercises range from straight leg raise, stationary bike, elastic resistance training, water exercise, and stepper-type devices (Fig. 15.3). Use of free weights and machines can be considered at this point if the exercise can be completed without causing pain in the injured area. The key is identification of exercises

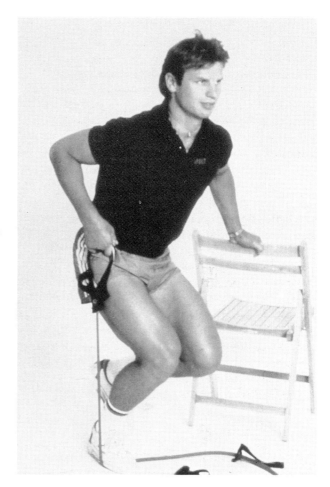

Fig. 15.3 Sport Cord single knee dip exercise.

which do not cause pain. Flexibility with quadriceps and hamstring stretching is included. These are generally static stretches. Use of simple modalities such as icing after exercise can be helpful during this period. At the same time, footwear can be evaluated with particular attention to correction of pronation with the use of foot beds. Our approach is to attempt to match the nonweighted arch with these devices, but not to overcorrect. Bracing with neoprene braces with or without straps may be helpful. Nonsteroidal anti-inflammatory drugs are used during this stage, but care should be taken not to create abdominal complaints. Side-effects should be anticipated and appreciated.

If this series of treatments is unsuccessful, then formal physical therapy, the second stage of treatment, should commence. This includes supervision of exercise modalities such as ultrasound, electrostimulation, iontophoresis, and phonophoresis.

As improvement occurs, the resumption of sport-specific exercises can begin. This includes elastic resistance exercise, increased cycling and increased water resistance with specific deep-water running.

If the problem fails to respond to these nonoperative measures, then surgical intervention may be necessary. This should occur only after a thoughtful attempt at nonoperative treatment.

Operative treatment

If nonoperative measures fail, surgical procedures are available to address these problems. For patellar tendinitis or quadriceps tendinitis, the average time to surgical intervention has been approximately 1 year in the author's practice. Thus, exhaustive attempts at nonoperative treatment have been tried.

With chondromalacia or plica problems, the nonoperative period is less, but surgery should not be initiated until nonoperative measures are exhausted. The exact time interval is variable, but generally rehabilitative measures should be used until the patient plateaus on functional testing.

Once a plateau has been reached, a surgical approach to the problem should be considered. In general, the least extensive surgical procedure which has a high percentage of success is the procedure of choice.

The procedures available include arthroscopy with secondary removal of soft tissue plica; shaving of chondral surfaces; removal of loose bodies; and occasionally a lateral release, usually extrasynovial through a small lateral incision. The second level of the procedure is the lateral release with medial reefing. This can be done in cases where the lateral release has failed to correct an alignment problem, and the distal attachment of the patella (tibial tubercle) is not lateral with an increased Q-angle.

The third level of procedure involves distal realignment. This consists of moving the tibial tubercle (attachment of the patella tendon) medially, and slightly raising its position relative to the underlying tibia. If this is done, the fixation should be firm to allow immediate passive motion to 90°. This motion should be continued throughout the first 6 weeks passively while protecting the knee from violent contraction of the quadriceps or sudden extreme flexion by using a hinge brace.

Patellar or quadriceps tendinitis

The pain which occurs at the quadriceps attachment of the patella or the patellar ligament attachment to the patella usually results from tendinitis. This can occur in various stages, from minor pain prior to undergoing rehabilitation to disabling pain after extensive rehabilitation.

Nonoperative treatment

The initial treatment is the same as described for anterior knee pain rehabilitation. A critical aspect of this stage is to rest the injured area while strengthening the muscles around the painful spot. Since the tendinitis is usually a failure of the eccentric contraction system which accepts the load, eccentric contractions should be emphasized. The type of exercise can be done with manual resistance, elastic resistance, free weights, machines, or water exercise. A stationary bike, a concentric exercise source, can also be used effectively as it requires little eccentric contraction which could aggravate the problem. The author's preference is straight leg exercise, short squats against resistance (elastic), bike, and deep-water running in a wet vest flotation device.

Operative treatment

If surgery is necessary, two levels can be performed. The first level is arthroscopy with release of plica, shaving of grades I–III chondromalacia changes, and possibly abrasion or microfracture of grade IV. In the open part of the procedure, the tender area is approached by a small incision and then open fenestration of the tendon is performed, making longitudinal slits in the tendon through the sheath to stimulate a healing response. If the degree of pain is severe enough and the duration of treatment long enough (approximately 1 year), then a second stage procedure may be performed. This uses arthroscopy initially, then open central fenestration is performed through the tendon. If scar is noted in the posterior aspect of the tendon attachment, then it is excised by making a T at the attachment of the patella and excising the scar. The T should be no more than one-quarter of the tendon on each side, leaving a remaining one-quarter of tendon on each side. The T is then reattached to the patella in a freshly created raw bone bed, using suture pulled through drill holes to the superior surface. Rehabilitation is rapid due to the protection of the one-half tendon which is intact, but return to sports is delayed due to the need for maturation of the healing tissue.

Chondromalacia and plica syndrome

These two entities are considered together due to their similarity in symptoms and treatment, and usual concurrent existence.

The initial treatment in most cases is nonoperative. Occasionally in a high-level athlete where the problem is disabling and the athlete can pass all functional testing for athletic function, an early arthroscopy is performed, but this is the exception.

Nonoperative treatment

The same program described above for the rehabilitation of anterior knee pain is used.

Operative treatment

If surgery is necessary, it almost always invokes arthroscopic plica excision and shaving of chondral surfaces. If grade IV articular cartilage changes are present (raw bone), then microfracture technique or abrasion chondroplasty is indicated (Fig. 15.4).

The rehabilitation from arthroscopic procedures is rapid. Several technical features of the arthroscopy can be helpful. First, the plica should be visualized fully, including suprapatellar, infrapatellar, medial, and rarely lateral. These are better approached from a portal which is mid one-third patellar or junction of mid and distal third patellar. This allows for evaluation of the inferior plica by looking down at them and the suprapatellar plica by looking up and appreciating the presence or absence of the suprapatellar pouch. This pouch can be eliminated by a completely compartmentalized suprapatellar plica.

The surgery includes excision but an attempt should be made not to violate the underlying synovium, while leaving a small rim of plica and obtain-

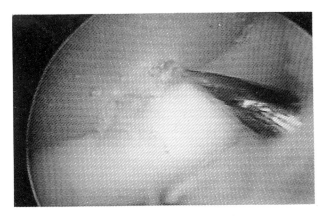
Fig. 15.4 Microfracture technique used for treatment of a grade IV articular cartilage defect.

ing hemostasis at the resection site. This is coupled with shaving of frayed articular cartilage and removal of loose bodies present. Postoperative rehabilitation is virtually the same as that used in nonoperative treatment.

On-snow injuries

Immediate care

Acute knee injuries are relatively common, both in Alpine racing and recreational skiing. The magnitude of the injury is usually worse as the speeds attained by the skiers increase. There are many ways that injury can occur to the knee. A common occurrence in skiing is when the skier puts too much weight on the inside edge of one ski as the other ski gradually diverges away from the affected leg. This puts stress on the medial structures of the loaded knee and may cause a sprain of the medial structures, or with further force, a total disruption of the medial ligament and posteromedial capsule, and possibly a tear of the ACL. Another common knee injury is created when the loaded knee is near extension and the skier falls backwards while the ski and lower leg are moving forward. This is likely to lead to disruption of the ACL.

Depending upon the injury suffered, the skier will have a lesser or greater amount of pain. In the case of a cruciate injury, the skier may experience a popping sensation in the knee, realize that something has happened, but be surprised to find that he or she can stand on the knee, perhaps with some difficulty. In some instances, the skier will attempt to ski down the hill and will make it successfully. With an injury to the medial structures, if it is a relatively slight sprain, the skier experiences some pain, but with difficulty, may be able to get up and ski very carefully down the hill. In most instances, in both of these injuries, the pain will be such that the skier will recognize that aid is needed, and not go down the hill.

Racers with a knee injury should be taken down the mountain on a toboggan by the ski patrol with the knee and the lower extremity carefully splinted. The ski slope is not the place for detailed examination and the ski patrol person should make only a general gentle assessment of the injury, ruling out a major fracture above or below the knee, or an open wound, particularly in an instance where the skier has hit a stationary object. Once this quick physical examination and history-taking are accomplished, the affected leg should be splinted and the patient brought down to the appropriate medical facility. In the medical facility, if there is a physician in attendance, an examination of the knee can then be done. It is somewhat easier to do an examination of the knee relatively early after injury because there is less bleeding and swelling, and that early examination may determine if there is laxity of the structures on either the medial or the lateral side, or of the ACL or posterior cruciate ligaments (PCL). After a careful physical examination, appropriate X-rays are performed if there is any suggestion of a fracture. One injury sometimes missed is an acute dislocation of the patella since the patella is usually relocated before the patient is even seen by medical personnel. The examination may seem relatively normal in that instance, but the lack of any ligamentous laxity and the presence of effusion and tenderness along the medial retinaculum may be an indication of an acute patella dislocation.

Much depends upon the amount of pain that a skier is having plus the skill and experience of the examiner as to how specific the initial diagnosis can be. In most instances, it should be possible to make an accurate diagnosis with a good history and physical examination.

Once the diagnosis has been made, a treatment plan must be formulated. If more studies are needed, such as X-rays or magnetic resonance imaging (MRI), plans have to be made to obtain these in the appropriate setting. This facility may be available at the site of injury or it may be more appropriately performed in the skier's home town. The knee should be protected during these initial stages while a treatment plan is being devised. In some instances, such as a first- or second-degree sprain of the medial structures of the knee, the splint applied may be all the treatment that is needed. However, it is absolutely essential to protect the knee from further damage while treatment is being planned and sought. In most instances, a protective brace or splint and partial weight bearing with crutches will be part of the initial care. Specific treatment modalities will be discussed in the following chapter.

Medial collateral ligament

Historically, the most common knee injury in skiing has been a medial collateral strain. This has been true since statistics have been kept. The severity of this injury can be graded according to the amount of looseness present. If the knee has sharp pain but opens minimally to valgus strain at 0 and 30°, then the injury is considered grade 1. If the knee opens up to 1 cm than the injury is grade 2. If the injury opens more and has no end point, the injury is grade 3. The grading requires a degree of clinical judgment. If the injury is accompanied by meniscus or cruciate damage, the treatment changes.

The steps in evaluation include history, physical examination, and imaging with routine X-rays and MRI if necessary. It is frequently difficult to obtain an adequate examination of fresh injuries due to swelling, muscle spasm, and tightness of the muscles due to apprehension on the part of the patient. If an adequate examination is not possible, then splinting can be performed and an examination completed later. If there is a need for immediate diagnosis, routine X-ray can be performed to rule out fracture or avulsion fracture and then MRI can be performed. If MRI is not available, then stress films may be helpful. This gives immediate information on the severity of the injury to the ligament. MRI is more enlightening, giving information on all ligaments, cartilage, and articular surfaces. This allows for immediate planning.

Important historical factors include the mechanism of injury, the area of pain, the presence of a pop with immediate medial pain, and a feeling of looseness after the injury. If the injury is acute, it is usually relatively easy to identify the painful area and examine it. If the examination is delayed, it becomes more difficult.

Treatment

Grade 1 injury

A first-degree injury can be treated symptomatically. This includes immediate exercise with a combination of stationary bike, one-third knee bends, water exercise with deep-water running, and a leg press. A functional brace that supplies medial protection and diminishes pain due to stretch on the injured ligament is used. As the symptoms decrease, more sport-specific exercises can begin. In skiing, this includes exercises which incorporate endurance, power, balance, and the repetitive up-and-down motions (concentric and eccentric contraction).

Grade 2 injury

Second-degree injuries include partial tears of the MCL. In these cases there is abnormal motion to valgus stress, and bracing is usually necessary. A functional brace which provides support against valgus stress is advisable, as it allows mobilization, weight bearing, and exercises. Then exercise is begun immediately with one-third knee bends, progressing to stationary bicycle as soon as symptoms permit. A Stair Master can be started early as well. Bracing in the functional brace continues for 3–6 months.

Use of elastic resistance, first for additional resistance during one-third knee bends and later for more functional training, has proven extremely helpful. The ability to simulate motions of skiing in this manner enhances the return to skiing.

Grade 3 injury

Treatment of third-degree or complete tears of the MCL have changed in recent years. The knowledge gained through basic science that these injuries can heal and even shorten during healing has decreased the necessity for surgery. In most cases where the other ligaments are stable, functional bracing can be used, supplemented with a similar program as described for the second-degree injury. The protection must continue full time for 6 weeks and then be used for sports for an additional 3–6 months.

When other ligaments are involved, repair and reconstruction are usually necessary. If so, the author suggests functional postoperative treatment as prescribed for nonoperative injuries.

Anterior cruciate ligament

Incidence of rupture of the ACL in skiing has increased dramatically in recent years. The possible explanations for this are discussed earlier in this chapter. Recognition of an ACL injury is usually obvious, but occasionally may be difficult. The typical injury is accompanied by a pop, although this does not always occur. A bloody effusion is frequently present, although not always. A feeling of instability is usually present immediately after the injury. As the early physical sequelae of the injury progress with swelling, pain, inflammation, muscle spasm, and capsular stiffness, the physical diagnosis becomes more difficult.

In making the diagnosis, history is important. A backward fall places the cruciate at risk. Another typical fall is the external rotation injury resulting in a combination of partial MCL tear with ACL injury. History of a pop accompanied by early swelling, although not diagnostic, arouses suspicion.

It is important to realize that an injury in skiing is frequently a multitude of injuries which occur at different times during the fall. In other sports, this is not the case, but in skiing, the lever arm of the ski, the softness of the terrain which allows the boot to get caught in the snow while the body continues to rotate, and the speeds involved may combine to create a complex pathology.

Another type of cruciate injury occurs during the slow fall where the binding may not be loaded enough to release.

The factors described above can create complex pathology which must be recognized. The examination should be completed with a suspicion that there may be injury to the medial structures, menisci, lateral and posterolateral areas, posterior cruciate, popliteus tendon, medial retinaculum, and articular surfaces.

The physical examination is usually diagnostic in the ACL injury. The single most important test is the Lachman test. This is done with the knee flexed approximately 20° and one hand holding the lower thigh while the other creates anterior translation on the tibia. The thigh muscles must be relaxed for this

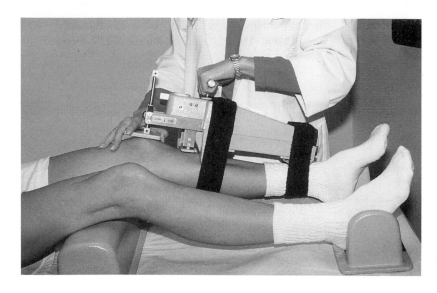

Fig. 15.5 Medmetric KT-1000 arthrometer used in diagnosing an anterior cruciate ligament injury.

test, particularly the hamstrings. Other tests include the anterior drawer test and pivot shift test. Results of these tests can almost always give the diagnosis in ACL injuries. Other helpful adjuncts are the KT-1000 arthrometer (Medmetric Corp., San Diego, CA), an objective measure of static stability in the anteroposterior plane (Fig. 13.5). In the acute phase, a negative KT-1000 test cannot be diagnostic. A positive test means a tear of the ligament, but guarding can prevent a positive test in the acute injury, thus a negative test does not rule out cruciate pathology.

X-rays are helpful to rule out fractures; the use of stress X-rays are helpful on occasion.

MRI can be diagnostic for a multitude of additional injuries that happen in conjunction with the ACL injury and can also provide information on the degree and position of tear in the ACL.

Treatment in a young athlete usually includes repair or reconstruction of the ligament. Controversy exists in the older athlete about operative versus nonoperative treatment. In the author's practice, repair or reconstruction is offered as a treatment alternative to older athletes. If surgery is performed, early mobilization is important. Commitment to postoperative rehabilitation seems more important than age.

Nonoperative treatment

Nonoperative treatment includes protected exercise during the first 6–8 weeks. This would include brac-ing and use of exercises which biomechanically protect the ACL and secondary restraints from deformation. These exercises include cycling, short knee bends, stepper-type machines, deep-water exercise, and progressive elastic resistance exercise. Machine exercise would avoid knee extension straighter than 45° and emphasize leg press and hamstring curls. Before returning to sports, the athlete should be competent at sport-specific activities.

Operative treatment

Many treatment choices are available for ACL surgery. The author's choices include complex repair with multiple sutures when the ligament is truly torn from its anatomic attachment. The procedure is actually a ligamentodesis where the ligament is fixed to the freshened raw bone bed and is supplemented by extra-articular reconstruction. A few cases can be treated in this manner. Most frequently, an arthroscopic-assisted reconstruction using patellar tendon graft with bone blocks at each end has been our choice. This procedure allows for early mobilization and rapid rehabilitation. The other alternatives include use of semitendinosus, fascia lata, or allograft. Each choice must be considered carefully prior to undertaking it.

Posterior cruciate ligament

Injuries to the PCL are rare in Alpine skiing. The history of a direct blow to the anterior proximal tibia with an abrasion in this area arouses suspicion. This injury usually occurs in a collision with another skier or with an obstacle. A second possibility is a combined injury where the MCL or lateral collateral ligament is torn and the knee rotates, abduction or adduction occurs, a deforming stress is placed on the PCL, and it ruptures.

The signs of the abrasion or contusion on the anterior proximal tibia and posterior sag of the tibia when compared with the opposite knee are usually present. The posterior drawer test can be diagnostic and the KT-1000 arthrometer can further aid diagnosis. Another helpful examination is the quadriceps active test. With the knee flexed one observes the tibia come forward in relationship to the femur.

X-rays are taken to rule out avulsion fracture. Neurovascular status must be evaluated due to the posterior displacement of the tibia into the popliteal space.

MRI can be quite helpful in diagnosis as it assesses the area of damage of the ligament. If the tear is proximal or distal, direct repair can be considered. In these situations, results have been excellent. If not, then our protocol is to treat the patient in extension for 6 weeks, allowing passive flexion in the prone position out of the brace. After this, rehabilitation focuses on the quadriceps as isolated hamstring contraction and flexion creates a deforming force on the ligament.

The rehabilitation continues with stationary bicycle, deep-water running, and an elastic resistance program, progressing to sport-specific exercises in 3–6 months. Functional braces, although not ideal, may be used to prevent hyperextension and direct blows to the anterior proximal tibia.

Medial compartment degeneration has been reported with persistent posterior instability, and should be anticipated. Yearly bone scans can be helpful in this diagnosis.

If reconstruction is necessary, a patellar tendon graft is preferred. PCL reconstruction is much less predictable than ACL reconstruction and thus there is less pressure to perform immediate reconstructive procedures.

Knee dislocation

Knee dislocation is a rare consequence of Alpine skiing. When it occurs, early diagnosis must be made and immediate evacuation from the ski slope be accomplished. The initial attention should be directed toward the neurovascular complications which can accompany this dislocation. Generally, closed reduction should be preformed immediately. Neurovascular status should be checked pre- and post-reduction, and usually an arteriogram is performed to assess regional circulation. The emergency room evaluation should be complete and all neurovascular status reported.

Once the neurovascular status is determined, some success can be attained with delayed surgery, assuming that reduction can be accomplished closed. If stability is retained after reduction, short range continuous passive motion (CPM) is used (30–60°). As the swelling resolves and the neurovascular status is clear after 3–7 days, then open reduction can be accomplished. Excellent results can be attained in skiers with initial reconstruction and careful anatomic repair of all torn ligaments. All meniscus tears should also been repaired. With this combination of early reduction, delayed repair and postoperative mobilization, we have returned many athletes with this injury to competitive sports.

Tibial plateau fracture

Tibial plateau fractures are uncommon injuries in skiing. They are usually the result of a collision. The initial approach should be to assure satisfactory neurovascular status. If present, definitive diagnosis can be made. Radiographic examination can be misleading, and diagnosis frequently requires a tomogram, computerized tomography (CT) scan, or occasionally MRI.

Once the severity of the fracture and the status of the ligament and the cartilage has been assessed, then definitive care can be undertaken. If the displacement or depression is slight, then early motion and bracing can be utilized. This is usually accompanied by non-weight bearing for about 6–8 weeks. If the displacement is unacceptable, then surgery should be performed arthroscopically, open or in combination. Near-perfect anatomic reduction in the weight-bearing area is the goal, and fixation should be rigid enough to allow early motion. Bone grafting with cancellous bone is usually necessary if there is depression of the joint surface.

Postoperative treatment with nonweight bearing is usually used due to the irregularity of the joint surfaces and damage to the articular cartilage. Continuous passive motion is a useful adjunct. Mobilization with spinning on a stationary bike without resistance or swimming are useful during early rehabilitation. Avoidance of impact on the joint surface is helpful.

Conclusion

Knee injuries are frequent in Alpine skiing. It is important to perform adequate assessment and provide a treatment program which is appropriate to the patient's requirements. With this rationale, it is usually possible to return a skier with an injured knee to skiing. If not, then the patient should be guided toward other forms of exercise which can replace the sport of skiing.

Recommended reading

Johnson, R.J., Ettlinger, C.F. & Jasper, E.S. (1989) Skier injury trends. In Johnson, R.J., Mote, C.D. & Binet, M.H. (eds) *Skiing Trauma and Safety: Seventh International Symposium*. Philadelphia: American Society for Testing and Materials, pp. 25–31.

National Alpine Staff (eds) (1985) *United States Ski Team Alpine Training Manual*. Park City, Utah: National Alpine Staff.

Steadman, J.R., Forster, R.S. & Silfverskiold, J.P. (1989) Rehabilitation of the knee. *Clin. Sports Med.* **8**:606–627.

Torg, J.S., Conrad, W. & Kalen, V. (1976) Clinical diagnosis of anterior cruciate ligament instability in the athlete. *Am. J. Sports Med.* **4(2)**:84–93.

Chapter 16

Leg

The lower leg is often injured as a result of skiing, and the most serious of such injuries is a fractured tibia (Fig. 16.1). Fractures of the fibula are much less important except when they occur as part of a complex fracture at the ankle. The tibia is a large and strong bone, and thus it takes a great deal of force and misdirected energy to cause a tibial fracture. While any significant direct force may cause a tibial fracture, it is usually rotation or angulation with force which causes the tibia to break. What usually happens is that the leg is broken because the foot is trapped by the ski and binding for at least a period of time and as the ski, foot, and binding go in one direction, the body goes in a different direction. The resultant force, usually rotatory or angular, causes the tibial fracture.

There are many aspects to consider as causes of tibial fractures. One is speed. This poses a particular problem in racing since the object is to go fast and get to the finish line more quickly than one's competitor.

$$\text{Energy} = \frac{\text{mass} \times \text{velocity}^2}{2}.$$

It is when energy is applied in the wrong way that a fracture or a significant soft tissue injury results. The following equation shows the problem of increased speed in racing. As an example, a 67.5 kg male skiing at 64.4 km/h produces energy equal to $67.5 \times 64.4 \times 64.4$ divided by 2 which equals 139 973.4. The same 67.5 kg male skiing at only 32.2 km/h results in an energy force of 34 993.4 ($67.5 \times 32.2 \times 32.2$ divided by 2). The magnitude of force is considerably less with the lower speed. Conversely, as he increases the speed, the amount of energy generated and available to cause problems is increased dramatically. Clearly, it becomes important to the ski racer to maintain good ski control and not to fall and thus avoid significant injury from the forces generated.

While most tibial fractures occur as the result of a twisting injury to the lower extremity, they can occur secondary to a collision as when the skier hits another object such as a lift tower or another skier. This second cause of injury, direct trauma, is less likely than indirect, but collisions combined with excessive speed can cause severe injury, and most collision injuries do result from high speed.

The pattern of ski injuries has changed dramatically during the past 25 years. Nowhere is this more evident than in injuries of the lower extremities. The combination of high stiff boots and effective release bindings has decreased the incidence of tibial fractures particularly in recreational skiing. In a series studied by Johnson and his co-workers the incidence of tibial fractures in recreational skiers was 4.9% and was declining rapidly over a 10-year period.

Many tibial fractures occur at high speeds, but they are possible at lower speeds when a skier falls, particularly with a twisting type of injury, with either a failure to release or a slow release from the ski binding. These injuries which are called lower extremity equipment-related (LEER) injuries have gradually diminished during the past decade because of equipment changes allowing quicker release.

Looking at the incidence of tibial fractures indicates how important it is to have good release bindings in proper working order. The authors of this book obviously believe in release bindings. However, it is not our purpose to recommend any particular brand of binding. There are many on the market which have been around for years, and most are constantly being modified and improved. Multi-directional release bindings are available and should be the choice. Information is readily available to skiers and ski racers in shops and in skiing magazines which each year devote a great deal of discussion to release bindings. All bindings should be installed and adjusted by a licensed technician to be effective. At the highest levels of ski racing the bindings will be adjusted by coaches, skiers, and technicians, all of whom have considerable experience. At the lower levels of ski racing the same expertise is needed but is not always available. It is relatively common to have a binding adjusted nicely at the beginning of the season and at the time of the first tumble the racer then decides to tighten the binding. For some peculiar reason it seems as if all racers can recount horror stories about having

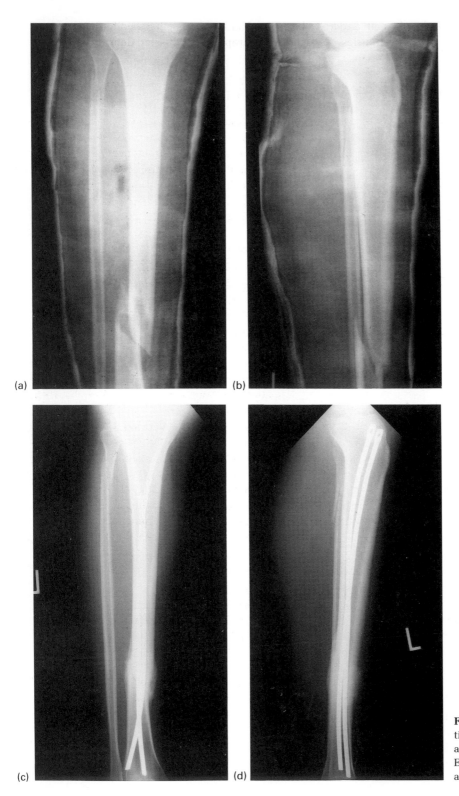

(a)

(b)

(c)

(d)

Fig. 16.1 Radiograms of an oblique tibial fracture: (a) anteroposterior view and (b) lateral view. After fixation with Ender nails: (c) anteroposterior view, and (d) lateral view.

had an early release which has resulted in a fall and a possible injury. While granting that certain injuries and falls may occur due to premature binding release, far more injuries occur as a result of bindings that were set too tightly and did not release when they should have.

Immediate care

In the vast majority of cases of tibial or fibular fracture, the skier is well aware that there has been a serious injury. The skier will either have heard or felt a crack, experiences instant, relatively severe pain, and usually presumes that a fracture has occurred. The immediate treatment of any fracture is important, and the tibial fracture is dealt with specifically.

Suspected tibial or fibular fractures should be treated as if they are real fractures. It is far better to splint and carefully handle 50 patients without one fracture than to poorly handle one and convert a simple fracture into an open fracture or into a potentially more serious one. The skier should be made comfortable and prevented from getting too cold while the patrol is summoned. The patrol will splint the leg carefully in one of the commercially available splints or failing that, improvise something to cushion and cradle the leg and then the skier will be transported to the most readily available facility for X-rays. Any suspected tibial or fibular fracture may be X-rayed while the leg is still in the splint, even with the boot on. Alternatively, the boot and splint may be carefully removed by skilled personnel who are aware of the probability of fracture and the consequences of moving the leg. X-rays are taken in two planes; anteroposterior and lateral. Once the diagnosis is confirmed, treatment possibilities are considered.

Few ski-related tibial fractures result in open wounds. The presence of an open wound changes the immediate treatment and may change the definitive treatment of a tibial fracture. If the skin is barely broken by what appears to be a small puncture wound produced by the bone breaking through the skin, it can be cleansed and the tibia treated the same as if it were occurring with a closed injury. If, on the other hand, it is a large wound with jagged edges and damage to the surrounding soft tissue and skin, this requires radically different treatment. All wounds must then be covered and immediately cared for in a hospital setting by proper cleansing and debridement.

Fracture treatment

The basic precepts for tibial fracture treatment are simple. How one accomplishes these precepts may be more difficult and lead to differences of opinion. The idea is to put the tibial fracture fragments in as near an anatomic position as possible and hold them there, either by a cast or a fixation device, until healing is completed. The average healing time for most tibial fractures is 15–16 weeks. In fractures which are relatively undisplaced such as a spiral fracture as is often seen in skiing, healing time will be shorter. For years, physicians considered bony union of a fracture the first priority and concentrated on that while giving less attention to the soft tissue. However, in the past several decades, equal attention has been given to the soft tissues of the leg and function of the leg itself. Rehabilitation of the muscles and joints of the leg is now started much earlier than several decades ago.

Most tibial fractures can be reduced by applying traction to the foot and lower leg and gradually realigning the fragments. Generally, the patient needs to be sedated with some intramuscular or intravenous medication and, particularly if the reduction is performed relatively soon after the fracture has occurred, a good reduction should be obtained. Usually a long leg cast can be applied while the leg and fracture fragments are held in position. There must be no rotation allowed at the fracture site. Rotation is a clinical judgment whereas position and angulation of the fracture can be seen both clinically and on X-rays. Most doctors prefer to apply a long leg cast initially with the knee in only a few degrees of flexion. It is now standard treatment in most tibial fractures to allow early protected weight bearing which is performed much more easily with the knee near extension as opposed to more flexion.

Following the closed reduction, anteroposterior and lateral X-rays are taken to determine the position of the fracture fragments. If the position is satisfactory, the patient may be given crutches and instructed on how to start weight-bearing gradually over the course of the next few days. The patient would be expected to have some pain during the first several days and should be told to elevate the leg. Increasing pain, numbness of the toes, or any weakness or inability to move the toes either up or down makes it mandatory that the patient return either to the physician or the hospital emergency room immediately. This may be a real problem for all skiers including ski racers. Most fractures occur away from the home area. This means that the skier, before leaving the care of the physician, whether it is in an emergency room, ski area facility, or the doctor's office, must be given instructions as to what to do during the next 24–48 h to avoid any later problems, particularly those that may occur as a result of swelling of the leg enclosed in the cast.

Operative treatment of tibial fractures

While most tibial fractures secondary to skiing injuries can be handled by closed reduction and application of a cast, some would be best treated by surgery. Depending upon the individual characteristics of the fracture and the skills of the surgeon, the methods of internal fixation which is most appropriate will vary from fracture to fracture. An open reduction should allow for an anatomical reduction of the fracture fragments and an internal fixation device should be able to hold them in position while the fracture healing proceeds. In such an instance the internal fixation may also allow for quicker rehabilitation.

Internal fixation devices for a fractured tibia could be divided into plates and screws applied to the external aspects of the bone and devices which are put into the intramedullary canal. The advantages of performing an open reduction and internal fixation are two-fold. In many instances a good reduction of the bony fragments may not be achievable by closed reduction while open reduction should generally allow for functionally and cosmetically good results. The second reason for performing an open reduction and internal fixation is that the bone is firmly held by the fixation device and the rehabilitation process is started earlier and more aggressively. Depending upon how solidly the fixation device holds the fracture fragments, the patient may not have to wear a cast or may only have to wear a modified cast or brace. This, again, allows earlier rehabilitation particularly earlier knee and ankle motion.

The average healing time of a tibial fracture is around 4 months, but most ski injuries are healed in a shorter period of time. It is, however, the soft tissues, the joints, and muscles of the leg which frequently determine when the skier will be able to return to full activity. At the time of early bony union the leg is not ready to take the stresses of major physical activities such as skiing. The longer that the skier has the leg in a cast, even weight bearing, the longer it usually takes the knee, ankle, and subtalar joint to reacquire motion and the more atrophy there is of the muscles of the lower extremities. Early weight bearing in the cast is distinctly better than nonweight bearing with regard to the effect on soft tissue. However, being able to remove a cast because the bone is securely fixed internally presents a real advantage for soft tissues.

There are a variety of methods for internal fixation of fractures. The Swiss AO (Association for Osteosynthesis) group popularized the use of plates and screws and their particular method of fixation has proven to be vastly superior to previously available methods. It is one of the excellent methods of fixation now popular and probably the choice of most orthopedic surgeons, particularly in the short oblique fracture, which is unable to be accurately reduced by closed means, and in certain other tibial fractures.

Intramedullary devices to hold tibial fractures have been around for many years. After an initial period of popularity, they became less so and now again are being used more as the devices have become more sophisticated. Not all fractures of the tibia can be securely fixed with an intramedullary nail. The closer that one gets to either the knee or the ankle joint, the less likely it is that an intramedullary nail can be used. The intramedullary nails have their greatest use in the transverse fractures of the middle third of the tibia. In these particular instances they can be applied in a closed fashion which decreases the potential infection rate while still allowing the excellent fixation afforded by the intramedullary device. The use of the anchored intramedullary nail allows the surgeon to use them nearer the knee or the ankle joint and in some instances in which there is comminution of the tibial shaft. The major advantage of the intramedullary device is that the fracture site does not have to be opened. And with good fixation, rehabilitation can proceed almost immediately. However, the form of internal fixation or the use of internal fixation should be left to the individual treating surgeon whose determination will be based upon the fracture type, the circumstances of the trauma, and his or her own experience.

Rehabilitation

Rehabilitation of a tibial fracture starts with the initial treatment. If internal fixation is used and it is rigid, it is possible that no cast will be needed or that the external fixation brace may allow for free mobility of the knee and the ankle. In some instances it may be that external fixation in the form of a cast or a brace will be used for a period of time and then changed to either no device or a lesser one. Early weight bearing is something that should be aimed for and as long as the fracture does not involve the knee or the ankle joint it is possible in all but the most comminuted of circumstances.

Most ski racers will have enough strength in their upper extremities, provided there has not been other injuries so that the use of crutches to give protected weight bearing is possible at the beginning. Swelling and pain are major worries during the first week following fracture treatment, but soon become easily controlled. Even if the patient is in a cast, it is usually possible to start the patient moving the toes up and down and doing quadriceps and hamstring sets to try to maintain as much muscle power as possible. It is also possible, at the same time, to exercise the hip adductors and to a lesser extent the hip adductors. While the cast is on, it is not really feasible to be able to do anything in the way of aerobic training. Once the cast is off more aggressive rehabilitation is possible. Knee, ankle, and subtalar motion become the immediate aims. Both active and active assisted exercises with the help of a trainer or therapist can be performed at this point. Attention is also directed to strengthening the muscles starting with very light nonresistive exercises and gradually progressing, always keeping in mind the status of the tibia. Obviously, major resistance exercises should not be started until the tibial fracture has demonstrated healing.

However, during this time it is possible to start on some aerobic conditioning which could be performed with a stationary bike or water exercises. Water exercises using a flotation belt are also very helpful in terms of regaining motion of the joints and lower extremity.

The rehabilitation program for a tibial fracture in terms of lower extremity endurance and strengthening exercises is relatively similar to that for fractures of the femur and various methods of increasing strength including free weights, elastic cords, or various machines can all be used in the same way. It is exceedingly important that the skier not return to training or skiing until the bone is completely healed and has remodeled. At the same time strength of the injured leg should be at about 90% or better of the other leg before the skier is allowed to return. The question as to whether or not the plate should be removed before allowing competitive or recreational skiing is still a matter of choice. There is probably some increased risk of a fracture as opposed to that of a normal bone when a plate is left in place. The exact nature of the risk is unknown, though it is probably low. There is also some risk for a significant period of time of a fracture occurring once a plate has been removed. This would be in the junction of the normal bone and the bone that has been previously plated. There is some bone atrophy due to the shielding effect of the plate and it takes a while for the bone to regain its strength. In the area where the screw holes have been, there is also, for a period of time, an increased risk. Eventually, those screw holes fill in with bone and should take part in the remodeling process that goes on throughout the bone. It has been the author's practice to remove all plates which cause any pain to the patient. It is uncertain, however, whether or not all plates need to be removed before allowing the skier to return to activity.

Anterior tibial compartment syndrome

A major concern for any skier with a tibial fracture who has had a cast applied is the possibility of bleeding into the soft tissue of the leg which may cause pressure affecting the blood supply to the lower leg and evolving into what is called an anterior tibial compartment syndrome. As pressure increases in the anterior compartment of the lower leg, it may affect the blood supply to the muscles controlling the dorsiflexors of the foot and toes, and this situation constitutes a medical emergency. It is both the bleeding from the fracture site and the exudation of soft tissue fluid into the muscular anterior compartment which causes the problem. The unyielding anterior walls of the compartment are composed of the fibula, tibia, posterior interosseous membrane, and the anterior fascia. As tissue pressure builds up in this compartment, it prevents oxygenated blood from perfusing the muscles and these oxygen-deprived muscles may become ischemic, non-functional, and even necrotic.

The most important clinical complaint for the diagnosis of the anterior compartment syndrome is increasing pain in the muscles of the anterior compartment of the leg. As pressure in the compartment gradually builds there may also be loss of the pulses in the foot, but that is usually a late stage in the syndrome. If one waits for the pulseless foot, it is likely there will be a long period of oxygen lack to the muscles and necrosis and loss of the muscle mass function will occur.

Patients always have some pain after a tibial fracture; even after the reduction and when the leg is in a cast. However, such pain should be controlled by medication and should not continue to increase. If there is increasing pain that is causing concern, the patient should see a physician immediately. If there is any numbness, loss of motion, or weakness of the toes, this mandates seeing a physician.

For the doctor the first step is to perform a quick physical examination of the leg and foot which takes a few seconds. Immediately, the next step is bivalving the cast and looking at the leg to determine the status of the tissues. If the anterior compartment appears tense or if the skin is erythematous and the area very tender, these are the findings of a likely anterior compartment syndrome. If there is weakness of these muscles this may be due to either residual fracture pain causing the patient not to want to move the toes or to an anterior compartment syndrome occurring. Usually the patient can be encouraged to dorsiflex the toes. If the patient cannot dorsiflex the toes it is presumptive evidence of an anterior compartment syndrome. Compartment pressures can be measured to determine if there is an increase in pressure above the norm. However, if there are signs of an anterior compartment syndrome the treatment is an emergency fasciotomy of the fascia over the anterior compartment muscles. This should be undertaken immediately. The fascia, the skin, and subcutaneous tissue should be left open and a delayed closure performed several days later of the skin. The anterior compartment muscles can survive without oxygen for approximately 6 hours, and any time after that will leave the skier with residual muscle weakness or total paralysis.

Chapter 17

Ankle and foot

The incidence of foot and ankle injuries has significantly declined in Alpine skiing since the development of rigid ski boots and the improvement of release bindings. Ankle sprains show the greatest decline of all the lower extremity injuries. This decrease in ankle and foot trauma is primarily due to the protective effect of rigid ski boots and to the reduction of friction between the boot and the ski.

Prior to boot and ski binding changes, 60% or more of lower extremity injuries were ankle fractures. All recent studies demonstrate that rigid ski boots allow minimal motion of the ankle and foot joints, thus protecting them against fractures or sprains. Injuries may still occur within the boot with rapid changes in forces over a small arc of motion. One disadvantage of rigid ski boots is that torque is transmitted to the knee without the normal compensatory mechanisms of ankle and foot joints. This helps to explain the increasing incidence of knee ligament injuries in Alpine skiing.

Three major injury patterns lead to fractures, ligamentous sprains, and tendon ruptures or dislocations in Alpine skiing and ski racing:
1 High- and low-speed twisting injuries (torque).
2 Deceleration injuries (bending).
3 Compression injuries (axial load).

Twist-related injuries are mostly caused by a valgus external rotation force but internal rotation can also occur. Ankle sprains and fractures are classically described as resulting from these types of movements. They can be produced if some degree of rotation is allowed in the ski boot.

Bending-related injuries are illustrated by forward or backward falls. They usually involve the tibia and fibula, in combination or as isolated injuries, at the top of the boot. The Achilles tendon may be ruptured by a forward fall with an anterior bending force.

Compression injuries occur with vertical impact when landing on a hard surface. The force compresses the ankle and subtalar joints producing tibial, talar, and calcaneus fractures.

Specific foot traumatic injuries are uncommon but pressure problems can be generated by ill-fitting boots. A bony prominence submitted to constant or intermittent pressure can react with an inflammatory bursa. Pre-existing problems such as bunions, dorsal spurs, pump bumps (prominent posterior part of the calcaneus), and hypertrophic or accessory navicular bones can be aggravated by ski boot contact.

There are 13 tendons which cross the ankle joint and transmit force from muscle to bone. Tendons have a tensile strength which is more than twice that of the associated muscle. They are more vulnerable when load is applied rapidly and obliquely. The most frequently injured tendons in Alpine skiing are the Achilles and the peroneal tendons. Vessels and nerves may also be compressed in a ski boot and lead to painful problems.

This review will cover ankle, talus, and calcaneus fractures; ankle sprains; tendon ruptures or dislocations and various compression problems.

Ankle fracture

An ankle fracture usually occurs during a fall with a rotational moment. This pattern combines external rotation, pronation, and eversion of the foot under the leg. Even in rigid boots, the talus can externally rotate and collide with the lateral malleolus. This force causes an oblique fracture of the lateral malleolus at the joint line or above and a tear of the deltoid ligament on the medial side or an avulsion fracture of the medial malleolus. Fractures of the lateral malleolus distal to the joint line generally leave the syndesmosis intact. When the fracture is proximal to the joint line, the syndesmosis has usually been opened with concurrent ligament tears. Torn syndesmotic ligaments allow talar subluxation and are potentially unstable lesions. They must be recognized and treated to avoid further complications (Figs 17.1 & 17.2). Internal rotation, combined with supination and inversion, is much less frequent in skiing. This mechanism may produce a tilt of the talus against the medial malleolus and an oblique fracture of the medial malleolus with a

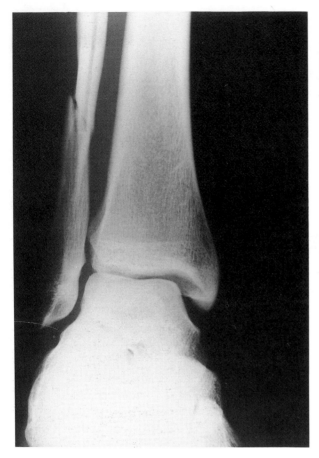

Fig. 17.1 Anteroposterior view of an ankle fracture. Fibular fracture proximal to the joint line; torn anterior syndesmosis allowing talar subluxation and torn deltoid ligament.

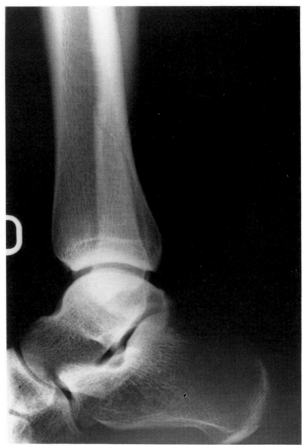

Fig. 17.2 Lateral view of the ankle in Fig. 17.1.

lateral ankle sprain or an avulsion fracture of the lateral distal malleolus.

Injury recognition

The patient presents with swelling around the ankle and bruising which can be seen laterally or medially depending upon the injury mechanism. Weight bearing is painful as is palpation of the fracture site. Tenderness is found in the sprained or torn ligament area. The diagnosis is confirmed by radiographs which include anteroposterior, lateral, and mortise views.

Immediate care

A soft bandage and a splint can be applied to immobilize the ankle. Rest, ice, and elevation should be

advocated before definitive diagnosis and treatment. An ankle dislocation, which is very rare, should be reduced as soon as possible.

Treatment

Anatomic reduction of ankle fractures is essential to prevent joint incongruity and late osteoarthrosis. Fracture reduction can sometimes be obtained by manipulation and maintained in a long leg cast. An initial satisfactory reduction in a cast may be lost after a few days when swelling has disappeared allowing a loss of reduction.

If the reduction is stable, we recommend the use of a long leg cast initially to control rotation at the fracture site. After 3 or 4 weeks, a short leg walking cast can be

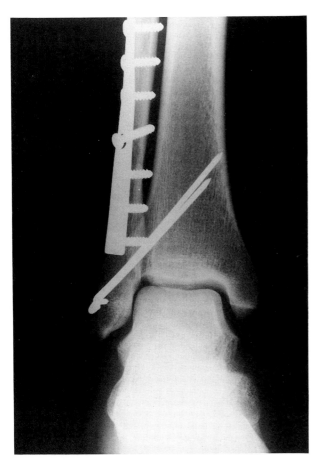

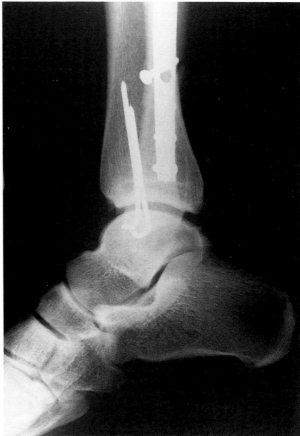

Fig. 17.3 Postoperative view of the ankle shown on Fig. 17.1. A plate has been used to fix the fibular fracture and Kirschner wires stabilize the reconstructed syndesmosis.

Fig. 17.4 Lateral view of the same operated ankle.

applied. The total immobilization is between 6 and 8 weeks. Undisplaced avulsion fractures can be treated in a short leg walking cast for 6 weeks. If the reduction cannot be maintained by a cast, then open reduction and internal fixation are indicated. The goal of the surgical treatment is to restore anatomical alignment and to provide stability, allowing early motion. The proper length and alignment of the lateral malleolus is essential to obtain a stable and congruent ankle. The lateral malleolar fragments are anatomically reduced and fixed with a small fragment plate and screws. Using the same lateral approach, the anterior tibio-fibular ligament of the syndesmosis can be visualized. If this ligament is torn, it should be repaired with separate absorbable sutures and stabilization of the distal tibiofibular joint obtained with two oblique Kirschner wires (Figs 17.3 & 17.4). A syndesmotic

screw can also be applied, through the plate, across the fibula into the tibia. The deltoid ligament, which is often torn in association with a lateral malleolus fracture, usually heals without surgical repair, provided the talus is anatomically reduced. Postoperative management consists of foot elevation for a few days. Active mobilization is started 1 day after surgery and walking, without weight bearing, after 3 or 4 days. A protective splint with ankle motion is used to reassure the patient. Early weight bearing protected in a cast is another option which leads to the same results.

Rehabilitation

After removal of the cast, a conservatively treated ankle fracture is usually stiff. Active range of motion exercises are encouraged several times a day. Weight bearing can be started as tolerated with crutches. Passive mobilization is indicated if the patient's condition is not improving after 2 weeks. After open reduction and internal fixation, early mobilization usually restores good function and stiffness is uncommon. Partial weight bearing is authorized after 2–4 weeks and is full at 8 weeks after surgery. Proprioceptive rehabilitation may be useful to restore the patient's confidence.

Risk factors

Ill-fitted and ill-adjusted ski boots are a major contributor to ankle fractures. Proper use of buckles can avoid uncontrolled ankle mobility and prevent accidents. Release bindings have to be properly adjusted by specialists. Their malfunction contributes to the injury risk. Environmental factors such as snow condition, temperature, wind, and visibility may also play a role in the accident incidence. Good ski equipment, proper use of it, and controlling speed are the best guarantees against accidents.

Prevention of injuries

Well carried out treatment, either conservative or surgical, should lead to perfect healing. Recurrence of ankle fracture is very rare. Complications, which can occur, include pseudoarthrosis, instability, and post-operative infections. Osteoarthrosis is the late outcome of post-traumatic tibiotalar incongruity or ankle instability.

Return to sport

Ankle fracture healing time is about 6–8 weeks when the reduction is stable. After 3 months, patients should walk normally and a full range of motion should be restored. Daily activities do not require full mobility and 10° of dorsiflexion are usually enough. In a modern ski boot, where ankle mobility is restricted, 15° of dorsiflexion are required to obtain a comfortable ski position. Running can be resumed after 4 months when good muscle strength recovery has occurred and radiographs have shown fracture consolidation. The patient may usually return to skiing after 6 months.

Pilon tibial fracture

This intra-articular fracture is the result of a compression force acting on the distal tibial articular surface. Such injuries are produced by a vertical impact when the skier lands on a hard surface after a jump. Normally, after jumping, the skier dissipates the energy by landing on the slope and continuing the downhill motion. But if the downhill slide is prevented and the landing surface is flat and hard, impact will occur between the talar dome and the tibial articular surface. The impaction of the talus upon the pilon surface may cause a comminuted intra-articular fracture. As discussed later, talus and calcaneus fractures can also be caused by the same compression mechanism.

Injury recognition

Intra-articular comminuted fractures produce massive swelling and ecchymosis which can threaten skin viability. Active motion of the ankle and weight bearing are impossible. Palpation of the tense tissues is extremely painful and tenderness is present over the fracture sites. Anteroposterior, lateral, and mortise radiographs confirm the diagnosis.

Immediate care

Elevation and compressive cold bandage should be applied as soon as possible at the scene of action. If removal of the ski boot is too painful, it should be delayed until arrival at the emergency room. Meanwhile the ski boot can provide good stabilization of the fracture and prevent swelling. A posterior splint is also useful to prevent rotation and bending forces on the fracture site.

Treatment

Surgery is required for most pilon tibial fractures. Open anatomic reduction and internal fixation is best achieved emergently according to the following principles.
1 Restoration of fibula length and stabilization with a small plate.
2 Reconstruction of the articular surface of the tibia and temporary fixation.
3 Cancellous bone grafting of the impaction fracture which leaves a bone defect in the tibial metaphysis.

4 Definitive fixation of the tibia fracture with plate and screws.

In some cases, swollen soft tissues contraindicate wound closure which has to be delayed for a couple of days. Postoperative management consists of elevation and rest for a few days. Early active exercises may start after swelling has decreased.

Rehabilitation

This type of injury usually requires a 12-week non-weight bearing period. Partial weight bearing can be resumed when bony union has been completed and radiographically documented after 3 months. Meanwhile active and passive range of motion is performed several times daily. Physical therapy may be required to assist the patient. Joint stiffness is not uncommon after such injuries and is correlated with joint surface anatomy restoration and permanent cartilage damage.

Risk factors

Avascular bone necrosis can occur in metaphyseal displaced fragments. Complications after surgical treatment of pilon tibial fracture include postoperative infections, stiffness, pseudoarthrosis, and late osteoarthrosis.

Prevention of injuries

Jumping and hard landing should be controlled and adapted to the skier's skill.

Return to sport

The healing time of a pilon tibial fracture is about 3–5 months. Normal gait is usually restored at 6 months and running can be resumed if range of motion allows 15° of dorsifexion. Skiing can be authorized after 12 months.

Talus fracture

As motion is almost impossible in modern ski boots, a talus fracture is very uncommon in skiing. Non-displaced vertical fracture of the talar neck can be caused by vertical compression. The same mechanism can also explain a talar dome osteochondral or "flake"

fracture. A fragment of the talar articular surface may be compressed against the tibial articular surface causing a subchondral trabecular fracture. If non-displaced, these fractures can be treated conservatively. Displaced intra-articular fractures require more sophisticated surgical techniques for an optimal result.

Injury recognition

Swelling and ecchymosis involve both ankle and hindfoot levels. Weight bearing and motion are restricted or even impossible. Palpation of the fracture site is very difficult to perform except in plantar flexion where the talar neck only may be palpated. Diagnosis is confirmed by anteroposterior and lateral radiographic views. Computerized tomography (CT) scan is useful to assess talar dome osteochondral fractures.

Immediate care

Elevation, compressive cold bandage, and nonweight bearing are useful. As for pilon tibial fracture, ski boot removal can be difficult and painful.

Treatment

Talar neck fractures in ski boots are generally non-displaced. To avoid displacement, these fractures are preferably treated in a long leg cast. The patient is kept nonweight bearing for 12 weeks and weight bearing can only resume when bony healing has been demonstrated in X-rays. The risk in displaced talar neck fractures is the development of post-traumatic avascular bone necrosis. The talar blood supply can be interrupted at the fracture site. This complication can lead to nonunion, bone collapse, and late osteoarthrosis. To avoid avascular bone necrosis, displaced talar neck fractures have to be treated surgically. With stable internal fixation early motion is usually possible.

Treatment of talar dome osteochondral fractures is a challenge. Nondisplaced injuries can be treated conservatively. Since casting of intra-articular fractures can lead to stiffness, early motion protected by nonweight bearing is preferred. Partial weight bearing can commence after 6 weeks. Displaced talar dome fractures can produce small osteochondral fragments which become loose bodies in the joint. Arthroscopic surgery is sometimes useful to remove such loose bodies and restore joint congruity.

Rehabilitation

After casting, talar neck fractures first require radiological examination to check bone union and avascular necrosis. The fate of these fractures depends upon the blood supply. Full weight bearing is normally authorized, if no complication has occurred, after 4–6 months. As early motion without weight bearing is advocated for talar dome fracture, rehabilitation is usually simple. If arthroscopic loose body excision has been performed, early motion and weight bearing can be resumed after 2–3 days.

Risk factors

Avascular necrosis is often described after talar fractures. This complication is followed by osteoarthrosis. A talar neck fracture is the most dangerous because it may impair blood supply to the body of the talus.

Prevention of injuries

As previously described avascular bone necrosis is a major complication of talar neck fractures. Nonweight bearing is advocated until that condition has been excluded. Axial loads must be avoided during early rehabilitation.

Return to sport

If no complication has occurred, normal walking can be resumed between 4 and 6 months after injury. Running and sport activities may be resumed later. Return to skiing may be expected after 8 months.

Calcaneus fracture

The incidence of calcaneus fracture is slightly higher than talus fracture. As calcaneus cancellous bone in children and adolescents is more resistant than in adults, calcaneus compression fracture is rare under the age of 15 years. Fracture mechanism involves axial loading and compression. Falls from significant height

or uncontrolled jumping and landing are always reported. Nondisplaced intra-articular calcaneus fractures may be treated with nonweight bearing and early motion. Displacement of the fractured fragments will affect the subtalar joint congruity. Surgery is therefore indicated for displaced intra-articular calcaneus fracture, to prevent late osteoarthrosis and gait disturbance.

Injury recognition

Calcaneus fracture produces massive swelling of the hindfoot and weight bearing is mostly impossible, except on tiptoe. Palpation of the fracture site on both sides is very painful. X-ray examination includes anteroposterior, lateral, and axial views. CT scan is often helpful.

Immediate care

Elevation and compressive cold bandage are important to control swelling. Weight bearing should be avoided and crutches advocated.

Treatment

Nondisplaced calcaneus fractures are usually benign. Functional treatment combines early motion with partial tiptoe weight bearing. Crutches are used during a 6–8-week period. Full weight bearing is authorized after 2 months.

Displaced intra-articular calcaneus fractures show joint surface depression. Open reduction and internal fixation often require additional cancellous bone graft. Early motion and partial weight bearing can be started after surgery. Late swelling may require further elevation.

Rehabilitation

Early motion is a part of conservative functional treatment and is also emphasized after surgery. The goal of early active exercises is to restore maximum hindfoot mobility. It should be achieved within 2 months when full weight bearing is resumed. Full mobility is often not restored after such fractures. Early range of motion is also recommended after surgery but weight bearing is more prudently resumed. Full weight bearing is authorized usually after 4 months.

Risk factors

Subtalar joint arthrosis and varus malalignment of the hindfoot are the major complications of displaced intra-articular calcaneus fractures. Gait disturbance, fatigue, and pain are often described by the patient.

Prevention of injuries

Persistent swelling is a common finding after calcaneus fracture. This may delay the use of normal shoes or hinder ski boots wear. Foot elevation is the best way to treat and prevent swelling. Axial loading and jumping activities should be reduced in case of chronic swelling.

Return to sport

With simple fractures normal walking is usually possible at 3 months. Running can then be resumed. Resumption of skiing depends upon residual swelling but should be possible 6–8 months after injury.

Intra-articular fractures require a longer healing and rehabilitation period. Normal walking is expected at 6 months and running at about 8 months. Return to skiing, which is dependent upon hindfoot pain and chronic swelling, should be possible after 12 months.

Ankle sprains

The majority of ankle sprains are due to inversion and internal rotation of the ankle as in other sports activities. External rotation can damage the deltoid ligament and the tibiofibular syndesmosis in specific cases. However, the incidence of these ligamentous injuries has been dramatically reduced in the past 30 years. Changes in bindings and ski boots design have been the major factor in this trend (Figs 17.5 & 17.6). Ankle motion is allowed when the ski boot is not tightly closed. The kinetic energy transmitted to the foot and ankle complex by a fall is extremely high. With internal rotation and inversion a primary tear of the anterior talofibular ligament is produced. If the kinetic energy is not dissipated, a secondary tear of the calcaneofibular ligament can occur. On the other

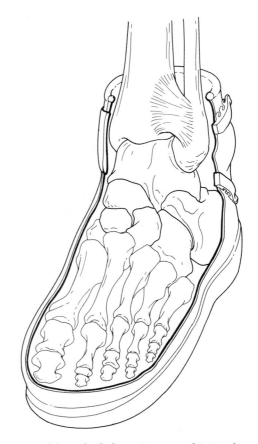

Fig. 17.5 Older style ski boot. Courtesy of A. Fasel.

side, external rotation can tear the deltoid ligament. In a recent study we have reported 10 cases of distal tibiofibular injuries in top skiers. All these patients sustained the same accident, straddling a gate during a slalom race. The rotational movement is extremely rapid and violent. The talus collides with the distal part of the fibula and tears the anterior tibiofibular ligament. If this external rotation continues further, tibia and fibula separate and the interosseus membrane and the posterior tibiofibular ligament may be torn. In competition, ski boots are normally well tightened but high external rotational energy can still produce tibiofibular tears (Figs 17.7 & 17.8).

Some ankle ligamentous injuries are associated with malleolar fractures. A deltoid ligament tear may be found with a lateral malleolus fracture. Syndesmosis tear can be combined with a lateral malleolus fracture and a deltoid ligament tear. Lateral ankle sprains can be found with oblique medial malleolar fracture.

Injury recognition

Areas of swelling, tenderness, and ecchymosis correspond to specific ligament injury sites and help to localize the torn ligament. Anterolateral swelling and pain between the distal part of the fibula and the talar neck indicate an anterior talofibular ligament lesion. Swelling and pain distally to the lateral malleolus are related to a calcaneofibular ligament lesion. Anterior swelling and pain between distal fibula and tibia, proximal to the ankle joint line, correspond to an anterior syndesmosis lesion. Involvement of the interosseus membrane is demonstrated when compression of fibula against tibia is painful. Swelling and pain around the distal part of medial malleolus indicate a deltoid ligament lesion. X-ray examination is mandatory to exclude a possible fracture.

Immediate care

Foot elevation and compressive cold bandages can reduce pain and swelling. An ankle splint can be provided to help reduce further pain and inflamma-

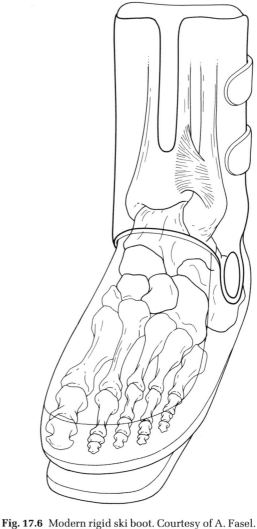

Fig. 17.6 Modern rigid ski boot. Courtesy of A. Fasel.

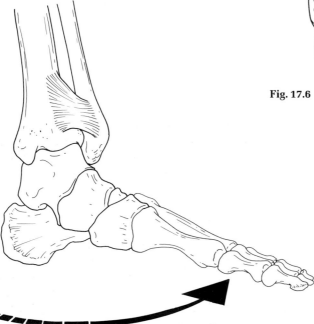

Fig. 17.7 Illustration of the external rotation producing a collision between talus and distal fibula. Courtesy of A. Fasel.

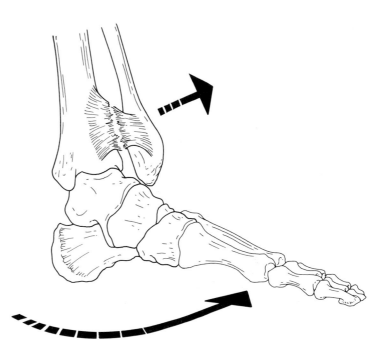

Fig. 17.8 Tibia and fibula separate and the syndesmosis is torn. Courtesy of A. Fasel.

tion. The patient should be initially kept nonweight bearing until definitive evaluation.

Treatment

Ankle sprains can be treated conservatively. We use an ankle brace which allows dorsi- and plantarflexion but prevents inversion and eversion. Weight bearing is allowed as tolerated using crutches. If initial swelling is severe, a posterior plaster splint is applied for 48 h. The ankle brace can be used after this first treatment. Usually ankle sprains heal in 6 weeks. At this time the ankle brace is removed. Progressive activity is then allowed depending upon the pain the patient has. Syndesmosis injuries require cast immobilization to control rotation. If the gap between fibula and tibia is abnormal, surgery may be indicated. The torn ligament should be sutured, using two oblique Kirschner wires to secure the reduction between fibula and tibia. These Kirschner wires can be removed after 6–8 weeks.

Rehabilitation

Functional treatment of ankle sprains includes early range of motion and active exercises. Rehabilitation starts and is accomplished during ligament healing. Proprioceptive re-education is advocated when weight bearing is resumed. Muscle strength can be restored with the use of rubber surgical tubing. This provides minimal resistance and is useful for early return of function. Physical therapy is also indicated after syndesmosis injuries. The same principles can be used.

Risk factors

Post-traumatic ankle instability is frequent when appropriate ankle sprain treatment has not been followed. Ankle instability may impair sports and working activities. Late osteoarthrosis is a possibility to be expected with an unstable ankle.

Prevention of injuries

When adequately treated, ankle sprains generally do well. Ski boots provide a rigid support, thus recurrence of ankle sprains is uncommon in skiing. The risk of recurrence is still present in other sport activities and prophylactic ankle bracing has been advocated by some authors.

Return to sport

Normal walking is possible with the ankle support. Running can be resumed after 6–8 weeks. As ski boots provide excellent protection, return to skiing is possible very quickly.

Achilles tendon rupture

Achilles tendon ruptures can be partial or complete. An acute rupture of the Achilles tendon is caused by a forward fall with forced dorsiflexion of the ankle (Fig. 17.9). This movement has almost been eliminated in modern ski boots and the incidence of Achilles tendon rupture has significantly decreased. Multiple mode release bindings also probably have an influence on this trend. Increased pressure within the fascial compartment of the Achilles tendon has been described with overuse of the gastrocnemius muscle. Poor blood supply which is caused by the swollen muscle leads to focal avascular tendon necrosis. This pathologic condition produces chronic tendinitis and can lead to rupture. The average age at which the injury occurs is 35 years.

Achilles tendon rupture may be treated conservatively but the high recurrence rate is discouraging. Many authors advocate surgical repair for optimal results in athletic patients.

Injury recognition

The patient reports a history of feeling a pop after a forward fall and presents with pain at the back of the ankle. The lesion is often missed because plantar flexor muscles can compensate for the deficient gastrocnemius–soleus complex. The patient may be able to ambulate and plantar flex the foot. A palpable defect over the substance of the tendon can usually be detected, but swelling of the injured area and into the tendon sheath may obscure the defect. A deceptive fullness at the rupture site, which is a hematoma, is classically found if the examination is delayed for several days. The Thompson test can demonstrate the Achilles tendon rupture and should be part of the overall evaluation of all ankle injuries. The test is performed on a prone patient. The examiner compresses firmly the patient's calf muscles. If the heel cord is intact, the foot will show plantarflexion. If the continuity of the Achilles tendon has been lost, the foot does not plantarflex. This is known as a posi-

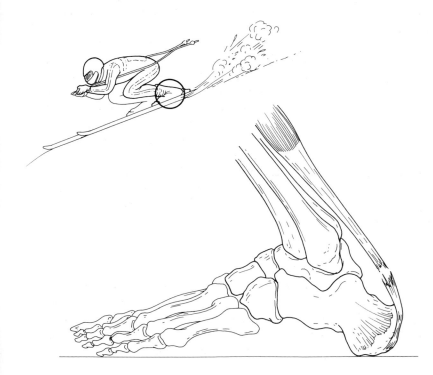

Fig. 17.9 Illustration of ankle forward flexion leading to Achilles tendon rupture. Courtesy of A. Fasel.

tive Thompson sign. Partial ruptures of the Achilles tendon can occur and will demonstrate a negative Thompson sign. If the diagnosis remains unclear, tendon ultrasonography or magnetic resonance imaging (MRI) may be helpful to assess the tissue damage.

Immediate care

A partial tear may be managed with rest and non-weight bearing. A posterior splint may be applied.

Treatment

Partial tears are treated conservatively. Immobilization in a long leg cast in relaxed equinus position for 6 weeks is usually sufficient. After cast removal a heel lift is useful for 2–3 months, to protect the healed tendon when weight bearing is resumed. Complete ruptures may be treated conservatively by casting in the relaxed equinus position for an 8–12-week period. For young, active, and athletic people, surgical repair is preferred. The operation allows an approximation of the torn ends with the Bunnell suture technique and absorbable sutures. If available, the plantaris tendon, left attached distally, is used to cover and reinforce the suture site. The ankle is postoperatively immobilized in relaxed equinus position in a posterior splint. After 4 days and the first wound inspection, an ankle brace is applied. This brace has an adaptable hinge which allows limited and controlled range of motion. Partial weight bearing is authorized. The brace is kept for 6–8 weeks.

Rehabilitation

After cast or brace removal, a heel lift is usually applied for 4 weeks. This shock absorber decreases stress on the injured Achilles tendon. The patient is encouraged to mobilize the ankle and strengthen the calf muscles. Active assisted stretching is then started to regain dorsiflexion. Full range of motion should be restored after 6–8 weeks.

Risk factors

Intratendinous steroid injections are dangerous and may lead to rupture of the tendon. Chronic tendinosis and peritendinitis are often misdiagnosed and poorly treated. Partial and complete Achilles tendon ruptures may result from these conditions.

Prevention of injuries

The incidence of recurrence is higher after conservative treatment than after surgical repair. A partial tear can also incompletely heal. Tendon strength may be insufficient to resist normal daily activities. Stretching and warming up exercises help to prevent new injuries. Jumping and landing with extreme ankle dorsiflexion should be avoided.

Return to sport

Normal walking is usually regained after 8–10 weeks. Running activities can be resumed at 3 months. With full muscle strength recovery, the patient may return to skiing after 6–8 months. Partial tears, with a shorter healing and rehabilitation period, allow earlier return to skiing.

Peroneal tendon dislocation

Acute anterolateral dislocation of the peroneal tendons from their normal groove behind the lateral malleolus is not a common injury. It has been reported in different skiing injuries as a result of a forward fall. A forward fall, while traversing the slope or making a turn, can induce a huge peroneal muscle contraction in the ankle facing downhill. The dislocation is produced with the foot in dorsiflexion when a strong contraction of the peroneal muscles tears the superior peroneal retinaculum. The incidence of peroneal tendon dislocation has been markedly reduced by design improvement in ski boots and release bindings. It has now become a very rare skiing injury. Cases are still recorded when ski boots are not correctly tightened.

Injury recognition

Dislocation of the peroneal tendons is often misdiagnosed because lateral swelling and tenderness over the lateral malleolus lead to the diagnosis of an ankle sprain. The history of having felt a "snap" or a "click" in the area of the lateral malleolus should alert the examiner. Swelling is localized over and just posterior to the lateral malleolus. Acute pain can be elicited along the posterior margin of the lateral malleolus. In some acute cases, the tendons are still dislocated and can be palpated over the lateral malleolus. In other cases, reduced tendons can redislocate with active peroneal muscle contraction. This test can be done in dorsi- and plantarflexion. X-rays have to be taken to exclude a fracture. Occasionally an avulsion fracture of the lateral malleolus is described.

Immediate care

If the peroneal tendons are dislocated, mild pressure will reduce them. Immobilization in a compressive bandage is applied before surgery. If conservative treatment is considered, short leg cast immobilization should be preferred.

Treatment

Reduction of the dislocated tendons behind the lateral malleolus and plaster immobilization is considered as the treatment of choice by some authors. As conservative treatment in a cast has shown a high recurrence rate, other authors recommend early surgical repair.

Early surgical repair is preferred because many peroneal tendons recurrently sublux after initial conservative treatment. Secondary surgery, moreover, is not always successful. The torn retinaculum can be easily sutured to its normal attachment. When a bone fragment is detached, internal fixation can be achieved with two small Kirschner wires. The deep fascia is then sutured over the repair. Postoperatively the limb is kept in a cast for a 6-week period. Recurrent dislocation of the peroneal tendons requires other surgical procedures. Retinacular reconstruction with a portion of the Achilles tendon, the so-called Jones' procedure, has showed good long-term functional results.

Rehabilitation

After cast removal, ankle active range of motion and weight bearing are resumed. Full mobility is easily regained but complete dorsiflexion can be delayed. Proprioceptive exercises with reinforcement of peroneal muscle strength are emphasized.

Risk factors

Inadequately tightened ski boots can induce many ankle injuries. Peroneal tendon dislocation can only occur if unexpected rotational mobility is possible.

Prevention of injuries

Recurrence of peroneal tendon dislocation after surgery is very unusual. On the other hand, conservative management leads to a high recurrence rate. Taping or strapping have not been effective to prevent recurrent dislocation of the peroneal tendons.

Return to sport

After 6 weeks immobilization, a 4–6-week period is needed to recover normal walking and full range of motion. Thus running is usually possible at 4 months. Return to skiing can be expected at 6 months. Residual swelling at the operation site can impede normal ski boots wear.

Acute and chronic tendinitis

In old leather ski boots, Achilles tendinitis was the most common cause of chronic heel pain. With the advent of high rigid plastic boots, this condition has almost disappeared. Various types of tendinitis may arise during running sports. As running is an important part of skiers' training, these pathologic conditions may hinder further skiing. Achilles tendinitis, posterior tibial, flexor hallucis longus, and flexor digitorum longus tendinitis may be recognized on the posterior aspect. Anterior tibial, extensor digitorum longus, and extensor hallucis longus tendinitis may appear on the anterior part of the ankle and the foot.

Injury recognition

Patients experience increased pain with activity. Tightened ski boots may be unbearably painful. On physical examination patients have tenderness directly over the affected tendon. Squeezing the tendon markedly increases this pain. Thickening of the tendon is sometimes observed. Pain usually decreases with rest. Ultrasonography and MRI may demonstrate structural anomalies in chronic cases.

Immediate care

Rest, ice, and strapping are sufficient to decrease acute symptoms. Chronic tendinitis requires shoe modification.

Treatment

Conservative treatment is usually sufficient for acute tendinitis. Rest, training program modifications, and adequate stretching may be helpful. In chronic cases a heel lift, orthotic devices, shock absorber, and corrections of all malalignment problems may be needed. Deep transverse massage, as advocated by Cyriax, followed by ice application is also efficient. Surgery may be required for a few patients who are unresponsive to conservative treatment. A chronic inflamed tendon may show partial tears, thickened areas, or nodules with mucoid degeneration and necrotic tendon tissue. Tenolysis with resection and repair of the degenerated tissue is performed. After operation a short leg cast is applied for 3–6 weeks.

Intratendinous steroid injections are avoided because of their weakening effect on tendinous substance. Tendon ruptures have been described after steroid injections. Some authors have reported good results with steroid injections into the sheath of the tendon.

Rehabilitation

Training program modifications, shoe orthotic corrections, and muscle stretching exercises are the most important steps in the rehabilitation program. Bicycling and swimming are encouraged.

Risk factors

Tendinitis can appear with overuse sports activities. Running on hard surfaces aggravates the symptoms. Intratendinous steroid injections need to be avoided.

Prevention of injuries

With appropriate medical advice and adequate shoes, patients should not experience recurrent tendinitis. Compression areas in ski boots can be corrected.

Return to sport

Gentle training may be resumed when all inflammatory signs have disappeared. Return to skiing is not contraindicated as ski boots do not hurt.

Boot problems

Ill-fitting boots can create pressure problems. These are the most common problems found in the skiing population. With well-adjusted boots, these situations should be avoided. Pressure problems are described with bone, nerve, and tendon.

Bone. Constant or intermittent pressure over a bone prominence creates inflammation. This irritative process may lead to bone hypertrophy with thickening of overlying soft tissues and adventitious bursitis. The points where contact pressure may arise are the anterior edge of the tibia, the malleoli, the posterior and lateral aspects of the calcaneus, the medial aspect of the navicular, and the 1st and 5th metatarsal heads. Some pre-existing foot malalignment problems may be aggravated by ski boots, namely bunions, dorsal spurs, and clawtoes.

Nerve. Compression can be seen on the dorsal aspect of the foot, particularly on the first toe. Sensitive nerves are caught between bone and rigid boot shell.

Tendon. The Achilles, anterior tibial, extensor digitorum longus, and extensor hallucis longus tendons can be irritated in ski boots. Local pressure on tendons create reactive tenosynovitis.

Treatment of all pressure problems is boot modification. Padding or relieving of the pressure on bony prominences can be adjusted easily by ski boot technicians. Unfortunately, chronic pressure problems are not always recognized and treated. Surgery may be considered if the problem does not respond to boot modification.

Modern ski boots have significantly contributed to the reduction of in-boot lesions. Therefore boot selection is important and the following guidelines have to be adopted:
1 Boots must be comfortable without any pressure points. Prior to buying, they should be worn long enough to detect any defect.

2 Movement of the foot within the boot should be minimized by perfect fitting. Proper size selection is important.
3 Stiffness of the boot should be adapted to the binding release setting.
4 Boots must be properly buckled while skiing. Loose boots are unsafe and lead to many kinds of injuries.

Recommended reading

Escalas, F., Figueras, J.M. & Merino, J.A. (1980) Dislocation of the peroneal tendons. *J. Bone Joint Surg.* **62A(3)**:451–453.

Ettlinger, C.F. & Johnson, R.J. (1982) The state of the art in preventing equipment-related Alpine ski injuries. *Clin. Sports Med.* **1(2)**:199–207.

Johnson, R.J. & Ettlinger, C.F. (1982) Alpine ski injuries: changes through the years. *Clin. Sports Med.* **1(2)**:181–197.

Leach, R.E. & Lower, G. (1985) Ankle injuries in skiing. *Clin. Orthop.* **198**:127–133.

Ruedi, T.P. & Allgower, M. (1979) The operative treatment of intra-articular fractures of the lower end of the tibia. *Clin. Orthop.* **138**:105–110.

Section 4

Nontraumatic

Health Issues

Chapter 18

Altitude

In spite of the fact that most competitive skiers are young and in excellent physical condition, they can be subject to the same altitude-related illnesses as those experienced by less physically fit and less skilled skiers. What is termed mountain sickness encompasses a spectrum of illness ranging from mild malaise to sudden life-threatening conditions. The major sub-classifications of mountain sickness are: acute mountain sickness (AMS), high altitude cerebral edema (HACE), high altitude pulmonary edema (HAPE), and high altitude retinal hemorrhage (HARH). The signs and symptoms of these illnesses vary widely and come about as a result of the body's inability, particularly the cardiopulmonary and nervous systems, to adjust to the demands of high altitude. To deal with these problems, an understanding is required of the physiological changes that occur at high altitudes.

The major physiologic stress encountered by a skier or any other athlete sojourning at high altitudes is a decrease in the oxygen content of the blood, which is termed hypoxemia. As one moves to higher altitudes, the atmospheric pressure decreases. The percentage of oxygen in the air is remarkably constant at all altitudes but the partial pressure of that same oxygen decreases in direct proportion to the decrease in atmospheric pressure. Thus, there is less oxygen available for the lungs. As the amount of oxygen available in the lungs decreases, so does the amount that transfers into the blood stream. There is, moreover, a tremendous variation among individuals as regards the response to this decreased oxygen.

Acute mountain sickness

AMS is not limited to very high mountains such as the Himalayas but is commonly seen in individuals going rapidly above 2400 m (approx. 8000 ft). Being physically fit, a requisite for ski racing, does not guarantee immunity from mountain sickness. In other words, mountain sickness occurs independently of physical fitness. Although it may appear that young people are more susceptible to mountain sickness, it may be that younger people exert themselves to a greater extent when training and competing at altitude than someone older would and, therefore, they are more likely to get themselves farther into trouble than the older person.

There is distinct individual variation in response to hypoxia (i.e. the lack of oxygen) which accounts for some of the variations observed at altitude. This seems to be a controlling factor in the spectrum of physiologic events known as mountain sickness. Any form of exercise such as ski racing makes the symptoms of mountain illness appear much worse.

The body's primary physiological responses to decreased oxygen content in the blood are aimed at maintaining appropriate oxygen delivery to the organs such as the brain and kidneys as well as to the skeletal muscles. Increases in lung ventilation (i.e. breathing) and cardiac output occur to enhance the delivery of oxygen and blood to these tissues.

A second physiological adaptation related to hypoxia is an increased production of red blood cells by the body which would improve the oxygen carrying capacity of the blood. This, however, occurs over a period of time and requires a number of weeks to become physiologically important. Despite these protective mechanisms to increase oxygen uptake, which should increase the ability to train and to race, there is a distinct limit to a person's ability to adapt quickly to the decreased oxygen pressure of the surrounding high altitude air.

The lack of oxygen which stimulates a person to increase breathing also causes the individual to blow out increased amounts of carbon dioxide. This causes the blood to become more alkaline. Alkalinity and the decreased oxygen interfere with the transfer of water in and out of body cells. Water tends to collect between cells (the interstitial spaces) and in the air sacs of the lungs (the alveoli). The body receives less oxygen not only as the result of decreasing oxygen in the air but because less oxygen is being transferred from the lungs to the body circulation.

AMS often affects the young and healthy adult. The

symptoms occur at altitudes greater than 2400 m (8000 ft) and come on within 24 h of arriving at altitude. Problems may begin after heavy exercise or simply after a night's sleep at altitude. Even previous stays at altitude without experiencing ill effects do not prevent the future development of AMS. However, it is true that those who have been at altitude a number of times without having trouble are less likely to develop symptoms, but this is not guaranteed. Alcohol intake seems to exacerbate the development of AMS.

Headache, restlessness, general malaise, poor concentration, and gastrointestinal disturbances are common complaints. Headache, in particular, is very common and may be severe. Inability to sleep is another frequent problem. Most of these symptoms are self-limiting and require little more than rest and adequate fluid intake for recovery. If symptoms persist and an individual is not doing well over a period of several days, it would be advisable to return to a lower altitude which would ameliorate the symptoms which would eventually be cured.

Avoiding AMS

Basic rules exist for the avoidance of AMS. A person should travel to altitudes slowly, a process termed staging which will allow for physiological changes called acclimatization. A reasonable rule for skiers would be to go up approximately 300 m (approx. 1000 ft) each day for any altitude above 2000 m (approx. 7000 ft). The problem is that many ski racers go from low altitudes to high altitudes quickly, and this makes acclimatization much more difficult.

The standard advice to skiers is to take it easy the first day after arrival and to begin with a light practice schedule. It is further recommended that skiers drink adequate water to maintain body hydration and decrease the body alkalinity. Dehydration occurs easily at high altitudes. More aggressive treatment would include mild to moderate analgesic for possible headache and a prescription drug such as acetazolamide (250 mg) three times a day. This medication, a diuretic, helps to promote bicarbonate diuresis to help overcome blood alkalinity. These medications should be given only under the supervision of a physician. AMS is not usually life threatening but would severely hinder any type of competitive athletic performance.

High altitude pulmonary edema

While AMS is normally self-limited it may develop into a more serious illness such as HAPE. In susceptible individuals, the capillaries of the lung become more porous, and this allows spillage of fluid into the alveolar spaces of the lung normally reserved for oxygen exchange. Because the oxygen taken into the lungs is now prevented from getting into the arterial blood of the skier, the individual becomes more hypoxic. The skier will experience shortness of breath and a rapid heart rate, and the skin may exhibit a bluish discoloration. Finally, the individual may experience agitation and confusion.

Laboratory tests may be non-specific but X-rays of the lungs will reveal patchy infiltrates which represent pulmonary edema, i.e. fluid in the lungs (Fig. 18.1). HAPE is potentially life threatening and early recognition and treatment are imperative. Rest and oxygen are key treatment modalities, but descent to a lower altitude is the cornerstone of treatment.

Traveling downward as little as 300 m may improve symptoms, but this should be accomplished rapidly. If descent is impossible, rest will be helpful, but it may not be enough. Breathing positive pressure oxygen

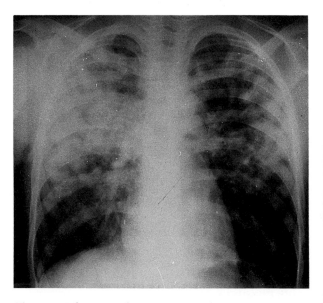

Fig. 18.1 Pulmonary edema as a result of exposure to high altitude. Courtesy of Altitude Research Division, USARIEM.

may be an interim treatment which is life saving. Recent evidence indicates that nifedipine is effective both in treating acute pulmonary edema and in preventing it in people who have had previous episodes of AMS.

High altitude cerebral edema

When mountain sickness worsens, it may result in a swelling of the brain known as HACE. HACE may be associated with dramatic symptoms such as severe headache, weakness, unsteadiness, inability to walk, and an inability to react appropriately to normal stimuli and events. Coma and even death are the terminal events of untreated or uncontrolled HACE. This constitutes a major medical emergency and the immediate transfer of the skier to a lower altitude is an absolute necessity. The administration of corticosteroid and oxygen may prove to be life saving in the interim period.

Visual problems

Visual problems at high altitudes may accompany many of the altitude syndromes. Engorgement of retinal vessels may be seen, and this may progress to retinal hemorrhage. However, hemorrhage does not usually occur below 6000 m (20 000 ft). This may be asymptomatic unless a hemorrhage occurs into the central area of the retina at which a blind spot will be noticed. If any visual symptoms develop, the only known beneficial treatment is descent to a lower altitude.

Respiratory problems

Another problem for racers who go to high altitudes is any type of residual respiratory disease. A person who has a respiratory disease such as acute bronchitis or asthma is already existing at a slightly decreased functional level. A severe cold or an asthmatic attack could make one temporarily more susceptible to a decrease in available oxygen. Moving to a higher altitude and engaging in vigorous activity such as ski racing with a respiratory problem, would certainly increase the risk of some types of mountain sickness.

Conclusion

Acute changes in altitude such as ascending above 2400 m (8000 ft) may seriously affect the health of the unacclimatized individual, particularly a skier participating in competition. Acclimatization by gradual ascent, limited activity during the initial 24 h, and adequate hydration are key elements to avoiding symptoms. Some people recommend prophylaxis with acetazolamide. However, most medical authorities hold that this is not needed for the vast majority of skiers or ski racers. Additionally, it's use is not recommended unless a skier has had symptoms on other occasions.

The spectrum of altitude illness varies from self-limited AMS to the life-threatening high altitude pulmonary and cerebral edemas. Failure to recognize early symptoms of mountain sickness may advance the individual into a life-threatening situation very quickly. Prevention with gradual ascent to allow for acclimatization and early recognition as well as descent when symptoms appear are the cornerstones of dealing with these maladies.

Recommended reading

Gray, G.W., Bryan, A.C., Frayser, R., Houston, C.S. & Rennie, D.B. (1971) Control of acute mountain sickness. *Aerospace Med.* **42**:81.

Hackett, P.H. & Rennie, D.B. (1976) Rales, peripheral edema, retinal hemorrhage and acute mountain sickness. *Lancet* **2**:1149.

Mountain, R.D. (1987) High altitude medical problems. *Clin. Orthop. Rel. Res.* **216**:50–54.

Chapter 19
Cold

During the past several decades, the escalating popularity of winter sports, including downhill and cross-country skiing, has led to increasing periods of exposure to cold weather. Just as all athletes have become more aware of the possible risks and injuries secondary to his or her sport, the recreational or competitive winter athlete must be aware of the unique problems encountered in cold weather.

Pathophysiology of cold

The problems in cold weather all relate to the conservation of body heat. Body heat can be lost to the environment by several mechanisms. The greater the temperature differential between the body and the outside environment the quicker the loss of body heat. Exposure to the air of any part of the body can cause loss of heat. Up to 50% of the heat production of the body can be lost through the uncovered head. In water, the body loses heat up to 26 times faster than it does in the air, which is one of the reasons that particular care is necessary during exposure to the damp environment during winter sports.

As wind velocity increases, it decreases the protective envelope which still air and clothing help to create around the body and this accelerates the loss of body heat. The rates of incidence of hypothermia (low body temperature) and of frost-bite increase dramatically as the wind-chill factor increases. Thus, wind poses a severe problem for the skier trying to preserve body heat.

The body attempts to conserve heat by several mechanisms. The primary method of conservation occurs by an unconscious restriction of the blood flow to the skin and extremities. This reduction in blood flow puts the skin and extremities at risk. It does, however, help to conserve the body's deep core temperature. At the same time, the body will try to produce more heat by increasing its cellular metabolic rate. Finally, the body can cause shivering, a method of increasing muscle metabolism which can increase heat production by as much as 500%. However, shivering is also an indication that the body is beginning to encounter severe problems with heat loss.

The body can be aided in its attempt to conserve heat by the insulation provided by clothing. A typical suit of clothes will decrease the rate of heat loss to approximately 50% of that of the nude body. Arctic type clothing may reduce the heat loss to as little as one-sixth of the unclothed body. However, should the clothing then become wet from either the environment or from perspiration, the heat loss of the same body could increase from five to 20 times what it would be with a dry body.

Injuries to the body from cold can be divided into two separate but at times coexisting responses, the systemic and the local. The systemic response is the condition described as hypothermia, a problem during which the core body temperature decreases to the point where even death can result. The local tissue response to prolonged exposure to cold can be categorized at frost-nip, frost-bite, and trench or immersion foot.

Hypothermia

The normal body core temperature at rest is very close to 37°C (98.6°F). In sickness, we often see an elevation of the core body temperature as a defense mechanism. However, during prolonged exposure to cold, the core body temperature may be reduced. When this core temperature drops to less than 35°C, the condition is termed hypothermia.

Causes of hypothermia may be either primary or secondary. Primary hypothermia is likely to occur in the winter athlete. The individual is normally healthy but, because of inadequate clothing or lack of protection, the body is exposed to severe cooling and hypothermia may result. Secondary hypothermia is that which occurs in response to another illness. Alcohol intoxication is a common secondary cause, due to its ability to disrupt the body's normal regulatory responses to cold exposure. Primary hypothermia may also be divided into immersion, which refers to exposure in water at temperature less than

16°C (60°F), and nonimmersion, which is exposure to cold air acting on wet clothing.

Hypothermia can also be classified according to the degrees of severity relating to body temperature as mild, moderate, or severe. Mild hypothermia refers to a body temperature between 32 and 35°C (90 and 95°F). Physical signs would include uncontrollable shivering, slow mental processes, poor coordination, loss of hand/eye control, and a distant gaze. Without complications, all persons should recover from mild hypothermia.

In moderate hypothermia, body temperatures fall to between 26 and 32°C (80 and 90°F) with accompanying signs of violent shivering and, in later stages, complete muscular rigidity. Other signs would include semi-consciousness, stupor, and pupillary dilatation. The clinical situation in this instance is very serious with the possibility of death being higher than 50%.

Severe hypothermia refers to body temperatures lower than 26°C (79°F) which results in a patient who is comatose and demonstrates irregular heart beat, decreased blood pressure, and decreased lung ventilation. At this stage, the possibility of death is exceedingly high.

Prevention

The best way to handle hypothermia is to avoid it. As the temperature goes down and the wind velocity increases, the chances of hypothermia rise. Moisture, light rain, and so on, increase the chances of hypothermia. Dressing to stay warm and avoiding getting wet are the primary steps to avoid hypothermia. Ski racing is a vigorous sport and that plus the production of heat by the body uses up many calories. A high caloric intake must be maintained so that the body has the means to continue to produce heat. If shivering is produced as the result of becoming cold this is an effective means of supplying heat to the body but at a major cost to the bodies stores of heat reserves and calories.

Hypothermia can easily result in death as a result of a multi-system failure in the body. Optimally, treatment should be hospital based and the patient taken to such a facility as quickly as possible. With mild hypothermia, assuming that there are no injuries, the diagnosis can usually be made with reasonable accuracy by recognizing the clinical signs: far away gaze,

stumbling gait, slurred speech, and shivering. The immediate priority is to raise the body temperature to normal. The idea is to get the victim out of the cold and wind as quickly as possible and into a dry, warm environment. Any wet clothing should be removed and insulation such as blankets, sleeping bags, or clothing should be placed over and under the patient. Warm sweet drinks will elicit beneficial shivering which will contribute significantly to the elevation of body temperature.

Once a victim has progressed to moderate or severe hypothermia, the condition is much more difficult and no procedures exist that can be implemented on the ski slopes. There is the distinct risk of cardiac, renal, and other complications which are associated with rewarming in the severely hypothermic patient. Again, the idea is to try to conserve the existing body heat and, particularly, to protect the patient from further heat loss. It is critical that the patient be transported to a hospital as quickly as possible.

If the individual is found comatose, lung ventilation should be assisted and the person should be transported to a clinical setting on an emergency basis. Once in the hospital, major resuscitative measures can be taken and rewarming can begin. It is important to remember that some people who have suffered from severe hypothermia may appear dead but have at times recovered. Implementation of the measures described above should be performed no matter what the condition of the patient might appear to be.

Local cold injury

Local cold injuries are often found in conjunction with the hypothermic systemic reaction. However, damage to the surface tissues, primarily the fingers and toes, may occur in connection with the body's attempts to maintain the more critical core body temperature. This local surface tissue damage can be organized under three basic headings: frost-nip, frostbite, and immersion foot. Under rare circumstances, eye damage can occur to the eyelid and cornea.

Mechanism of injury

As stated previously, the body's primary method of maintaining the normal deep body core temperature in a cold atmosphere is by constricting the blood vessels to the extremities. This results in a decrease in the warming blood flow and diverts the blood to the deeper tissues. Secondary to this phenomenon, the skin temperature can reach that of the ambient temperature. When temperatures are at or near freezing point, damage to tissues can occur by means of two different mechanisms. The first mechanism involves the freezing of tissues with direct damage to tissue cells. The second involves the indirect mechanism of ischemia from vasoconstriction leading to cell death from anoxia.

Frost-nip

Frost-nip is the mildest form of local cold injury and is commonly seen in the fast-moving downhill skier. It usually occurs on the nose, ears, or hands and represents a reversible blanching and numbness of the skin. Frost-nip can be completely prevented by proper clothing and thus kept from progressing on to frost-bite.

Frost-nip appears suddenly as a small, colorless or white area of the skin termed blanching. It represents ice crystals forming from water trapped in the superficial, dead layers of the body skin.

If frost-nip occurs, immediate warming of the affected area can prevent frost-bite of the living tissue beneath. One of the problems for skiers is that they frequently cannot recognize that frost-nip is occurring. Teammates or coaches may have to point out what is happening. In such an instance, protection of the hands or affected area or warming even by another person are usually enough to stop the process. The patient must then further protect the area or get out of the cold and wind. No living tissue is damaged in a frost-nip incident as long as the process is reversed immediately.

Frost-bite

Frost-bite is a common injury incurred in the cold which is exacerbated by wind. Superficial frost-bite involves damage to the skin and the immediate subcutaneous tissue. Blanching occurs followed by hyperemia and swelling. Upon rewarming, large clear blisters form on the skin as the damage increases (Figs 19.1 & 19.2). The individual must not tolerate numbness in fingers or toes for any extended period

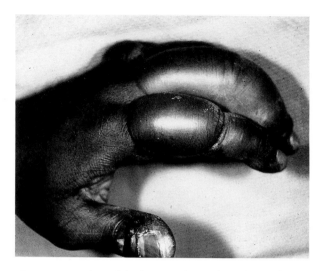

Fig. 19.1 Frost-bite of the fingers. Blisters form during the first 12 h after frost-bite injury. Clear fluid is a good prognostic sign. Courtesy of M. Hamlet.

because tissue injury occurs rapidly. Deep frost-bite involves the full thickness of the skin and even some of the deeper tissues including bone. In these severe cases, the blisters may be smaller and blood filled. The resultant damage which causes these blisters may lead to tissue necrosis and loss of body parts.

One important principle concerning the treatment of frost-bite is that no active rewarming should be initiated if there is a danger of refreezing. However, the normal initial treatment would be the removal of the skier from the cold environment followed by restoration of normal body temperature. The affected area should be rewarmed rapidly in a tub of water heated to 40–42°C (approx. 104–108°F).

Trauma to the affected area must be avoided as even rough handling of tissues may cause further damage. Frost-bite constitutes a true medical emergency and, therefore, hospital care should be initiated as soon as possible. The "old time remedy" of rubbing the affected area with snow or anything else should be avoided as it is clearly counterproductive.

Skiers and other winter athletes are constantly exposed to frost-bite. A person who has suffered from frost-bite to a particular area immediately becomes more susceptible to recurring frost-bite in that area in the future. This requires that the skier take great care to protect that part from any combination of cold and

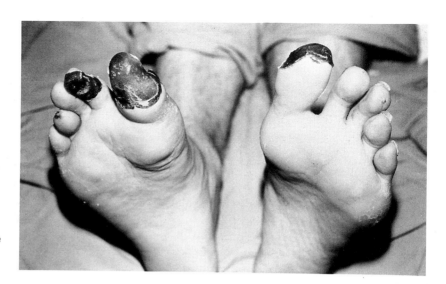

Fig. 19.2 Frost-bite of the toes 4–5 weeks after injury. Mummifying tissue is clearly demarcated and sloughing. Courtesy of M. Hamlet.

wind. Sequelae of frost-bite can include extreme cold sensitivity, vasoconstriction, and excessive perspiration in the area damaged. As with all cold injuries, the most important factor is appropriate clothing.

Immersion foot

Immersion foot or trench foot can occur in the cold weather athlete but it more commonly seen in soldiers or sailors exposed to cold weather and water. At temperatures near or just above freezing when the lower extremities are constricted by outer clothing, blood flow to the feet may be compromised. Long-term vasoconstriction along with blunt trauma of marching are common causes. Standing or sitting for long periods with wet feet produces this injury.

Initial symptoms include numbness, often accompanied by a tingling pain and itching in the involved area. This may progress to cramping and complete numbness of the involved area. The end result is often a discolored blue/gray foot with some swelling and decreased sensation. Liquefaction necrosis occurs which requires amputation.

The treatment of the skier with immersion foot involves gentle rewarming and drying of the involved area. Recovery may take several months and result in a foot which is chronically sensitive to cold. It is extremely important for the skier to keep the feet dry and, for this reason, woolen socks are extremely effective in foot protection.

Recommended reading

Bangs, G. & Hamlet, M.P. (1987) Hypothermia and cold injuries. In Auerbach, P.S. & Geehr, E.C. (eds) *Management of Wilderness and Environmental Emergencies*. New York: Macmillan, pp. 27–62.

Edlich, R.F., Chang, D.E., Birk, K.A., Morgan, R.F. & Tafel, J.A. (1989) Cold injuries. *Comp. Ther.* **15(9)**:13–21.

Grace, T.G. (1978) Cold exposure injuries and the winter athlete. *Clin. Orthop. Rel. Res.* **216**:55–62.

Heggers, J.P., Robson, M.C., Manvalen, K. *et al.* (1987) Experimental and clinical observations of frostbite. *Ann. Emerg. Med.* **16**:1056–1062.

Chapter 20

Sun

Recreational skiers look forward to clear winter or spring days when the sun is out and it is warm enough for light jackets or shirt-sleeve skiing. For the racer, sunlight may offer the advantage of delineating the topography of the race course and may soften the snow surface enough to hold the edges a bit easier. However, for all skiers, sunlight may present major problems. Foremost is the damage that sun causes to the skin. For years, people have actively sought out the sun to become tanned and "healthy looking," not recognizing the damage done to the skin, particularly over the long term. We now recognize that the sun's rays may damage the skin severely. This problem is intensified for skiers because of the background of large snow fields which reflect the sun's rays, constantly exposing the skier's ears, face, nose, and neck to ultraviolet radiation. Another consideration is that much skiing is done at high altitudes where the atmosphere absorbs less of the sun's rays. The intensity of light at 1650 m (5000 ft) is 20% higher than it is at sea level. Thus, the skier's exposed skin is exposed to more intense sunlight, both because of the white snowy background and the higher altitudes.

Light can be divided into several different groupings. Ultraviolet A is the usual daylight sun that we see and it is capable of penetrating glass and generally will cause light tanning. Ultraviolet B is present and predominant when the sun is very high in the sky around noon. It will not penetrate glass, but is capable of causing severe burning of the skin. While skin may be protected externally by clothing and other substances, it is protected normally by melanin, a pigment contained in the deeper layers of the skin, which causes tanning. People with dark complexions have more melanin in their skin than those with light complexions. People with Nordic coloring, i.e. those with light skin and blond or red hair, are more likely to suffer skin damage than those who have a darker complexion of skin.

Sunburn is literally that, a burning of the skin. The ultraviolet rays cause inflammation of the layers under the skin with reddening and even blister formation. This thermal injury is the same as one might suffer from a fire. There has always been concern about the short-term effects of sunburn, particularly pain, but there is less awareness of the cumulative damage to the skin. With sun exposure over a period of years, damage occurs to the underlying subcutaneous tissues below the skin. This causes thinning of the skin and a loss of the support structures which leads to the wrinkles which we see in elderly people and those exposed to the sun constantly.

Skin cancer

There are other sun-related problems, however. There is a high incidence of various forms of skin cancer in people with constant exposure to the sun's rays. One type, basal cell skin cancer, is a local growth, which may penetrate deeply, but can be treated by surgical excision locally. The second type, squamous cell cancer, is also treated by local excision, but has the capacity to travel to other parts of the body, although that is uncommon. The third form of skin cancer, melanoma, is malignant and if not caught early, may metastasize to other areas of the body and may even cause death. The 1980s have shown a tremendous increase in the number of skin cancers diagnosed, and this parallels the exposure that large groups of people have had to the sun's rays.

Skin protection

For the skier, skin protection comes either by clothing or by applying certain materials to the skin. The neck, ears, and much of the face are difficult to protect with clothing and should be protected by some blocking agent. Zinc or titanium oxide are substances applied to the skin which literally block the sun's ultraviolet rays from getting to the skin. However, they wash off rather easily which results in a loss of effectiveness. Most people now use sunscreens containing para-aminobenzoic acid (PABA), a paraaminobenzoic ester or cinnamate. These compounds actually absorb ultraviolet energy and thus protect the skin. They are usually combined with cream, oil, or alcohol and even perfumes.

Sunscreens have a standard protection factor (SPF) number which correlates with a protection scheme that is not well standardized. A sunscreen rating of 15 implies that you could be exposed to sunlight 15 times longer and get the same exposure effects as on the skin without protection applied. The higher ratings give higher protection. Moisture, such as perspiration may wash off these agents. Certain medication, such as antibiotics (e.g. tetracycline) may increase photo-sensitization of the skin and people using antibiotics must have high SPF blockers. Some people do become sensitized or allergic to either PABA or the perfume in the blocking agents.

The worst time of day for sun damage is between 11 a.m. and 2 p.m. when the sun is directly overhead. Even when it is cloudy, people are being exposed to ultraviolet radiation and must protect the skin and the eyes. A cool day and a light wind lessen the feeling of heat, and skiers may be less careful in applying sun-blockers. The lips have less natural melanin and may need several applications during the day.

Recommended reading

Howe, N. (1983) Skiing may be hazardous to your skin. *Skiing* **35**:91–93.

Taylor, C.R., Stern, R.S., Leyden, J.J. & Gilchrest, B.A. (1990) Photoaging, photodamage, and photoprotection. *J. Am. Acad. Dermatol.* **22**:1–15.

Index